COMPLETE INTERMITTENT FASTING

Complete Intermittent Fasting

Practical Guidelines and Healthy Recipes
to Lose Weight and Improve Wellness

Jean LaMantia, RD

Photography by Darren Muir

**ROCKRIDGE
PRESS**

For general information on our other products and services or to obtain technical support, please contact our Customer Care Department within the United States at (866) 744-2665, or outside the United States at (510) 253-0500.

Rockridge Press publishes its books in a variety of electronic and print formats. Some content that appears in print may not be available in electronic books, and vice versa.

Interior and Cover Designer: Brian Lewis
Art Producer: Megan Baggott
Editor: Natasha Yglesias and Claire Yee
Production Editor: Matthew Burnett

Photography © 2020 Darren Muir
Illustrations © 2020 Alex Asfour
Author photograph courtesy of Diana Nazareth
Cover: Kale Salad with Roasted Sweet Potatoes, Pepitas, and Raspberry Vinaigrette, page 122; Lemon-Lavender Muffins, page 118

ISBN: Print 978-1-64611-953-0
eBook 978-1-64611-954-7
R0

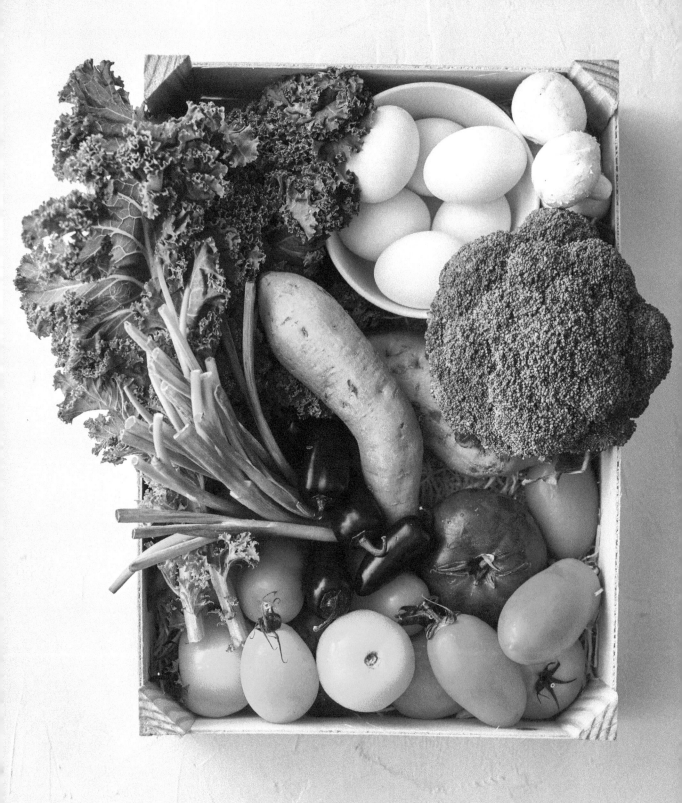

Contents

PART ONE

The Science

Intermittent fasting is an evidence-based eating program, although its roots stem from a blend of evolution, religion, and even politics. We'll explore some of the nutritional research on intermittent fasting and I'll explain the benefits, risks, and recommendations so you can get the most out of this approach for your specific goals.

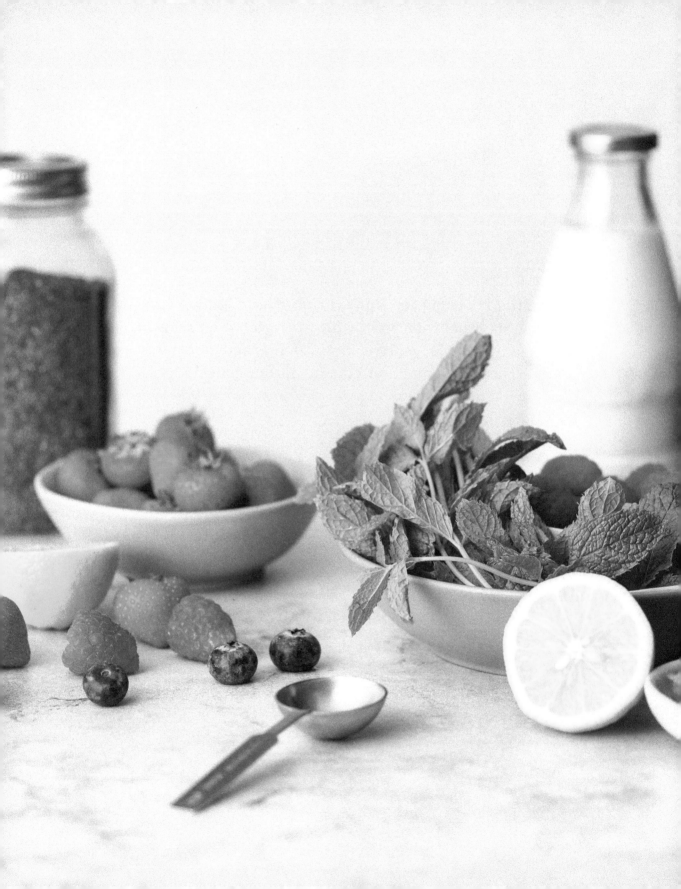

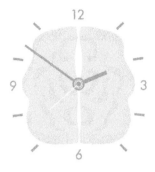

CHAPTER ONE

What Is Intermittent Fasting?

In this chapter, I provide the basics on intermittent fasting (IF) and cover the broad mechanics of how it works. I'll lay out the details and benefits so you can feel confident about fasting if you choose to practice it. I encourage you to digest this section (no pun intended), rather than skip ahead to the practical application because I think you'll find that understanding fasting is key to making it sustainable.

Intermittent Fasting Isn't New

Fasting has been around since early times. Our hunter-gatherer ancestors fasted, but this was because of necessity and availability of food, not choice. Many cultures around the world have developed fasting as part of religious observance and for medical purposes, too.

Ancient Greeks believed that eating food was a portal for demons to enter the body and were required to fast to prepare for rituals and celebrations. Praising the benefits of fasting has been attributed to biblical figures including Moses, Elias, and John the Baptist, as well as Pythagoras, the ancient Greek philosopher and mathematician.

Today, fasting traditions are still practiced by Muslims, who fast for the entire month of Ramadan from sunup until sundown, and Jewish people, who fast and pray for 25 hours during Yom Kippur. Throughout Lent, Catholics abstain from certain foods to honor Jesus's 40 days in the desert.

In the mid-1800s, Dr. E. H. Dewey wrote a book called *The True Science of Living*, in which he promoted fasting on the basis that disease develops when we eat more than our gastric juices can manage.

In more recent history, American physiologist Ancel Keys conducted experiments on fasting and published his book *The Biology of Human Starvation* in 1950. Medical fasting gave way to ketogenic diets for the treatment of epilepsy and management of obesity.

So, although interest in intermittent fasting continues today, there exists an almost 2,500-year-old practice behind it! We can keep this history in mind while refining and individualizing fasting to maximize the benefits based on our goals and current scientific research.

How and Why It Works

Three key mechanisms explain how and why intermittent fasting works. The first is based on a system of internal clocks inside our brain and throughout our body, which includes the master circadian clock and peripheral clocks.

The Master Clock

The master (circadian) clock is a small part of the brain that controls hormones and neurons based on input it receives from the eyes regarding whether it's day or night. Based on light levels, the master clock determines which hormones to release and which neurons to signal. For example, as light levels fall in the evening, it releases melatonin, a hormone to help us fall asleep.

The Peripheral Clocks

In addition to the master clock, there are also peripheral clocks in our cells. Unlike the master clock, whose main switch is light and dark, the main switch for these peripheral clocks is *eating*. These peripheral clocks have a big impact on the body's metabolism.

Peripheral clocks affect our hormones. Eating food late at night may reset these peripheral clocks and lead to changes in energy storage. Insulin plays an important role here. If your goal is to lose weight, it's not good to have higher circulating levels of insulin in the evening. Fasting regimens that limit energy intake in the evening make the body align with the light-dark cycle, leading to improved body weight regulation. In addition, our bodies naturally experience more insulin resistance in the evenings and eating at night means your blood sugar and insulin will stay higher longer.

The Microbiome

The second key mechanism to explain how and why intermittent fasting works is the gastrointestinal (GI) microbiome. An important part of the GI tract is the small intestine, which is home to a vast number of live bacteria, collectively known as the microbiome, microbiota, GI flora, or gut flora.

The gut microbiome consists of the largest number and most diverse population of bacteria in the entire body. This microbiome has its own circadian rhythm, which becomes disrupted when eating and fasting deviate from a normal day/night pattern and when an individual is obese.

When you're overweight, the makeup of the microbiome changes so you absorb more calories from your food, contributing to more obesity. Restoring a normal eating and fasting routine to match day/night helps restore the normal makeup of bacteria in the gut. In addition, an extended fast can reduce the permeability of the gut and prevent leakage of endotoxins, which contributes to inflammation.

LIFESTYLE BEHAVIORS

The final important mechanism behind successful intermittent fasting involves two key lifestyle behaviors: the ability to consume fewer calories and improved sleep. Both behaviors have been shown to contribute positively to weight loss. Research has demonstrated that a 14-hour fast reduces calorie intake and weight and improves sleep, hunger control, and energy levels.

How Insulin, Glucose, and Hormones Are Supposed to Work

When it comes to intermittent fasting, there are some key biological players. We'll discuss how these components normally work in the body.

Insulin is a hormone. Think of insulin as a key. Once blood sugar goes up, insulin is released into the bloodstream, looking for a keyhole (cell receptor). When it finds the keyhole and locks in, the cell opens and the sugar enters. Then the cell can use that sugar for energy.

Glucose is a single sugar. When you eat any type of carbohydrate, the body breaks down the food into its smallest component: glucose. It then passes through the lining of the small intestine and enters the bloodstream. The rise in blood sugar signals the pancreas to release insulin, which will find the cell receptor to let in the sugar.

It's normal after eating to have a rise in blood sugar followed by a rise in insulin, then a fall in blood sugar and a fall in insulin. Our blood sugar levels fluctuate throughout the day. The lowest blood sugar occurs first thing in the morning before eating (called a fasting blood sugar). The normal fasting blood sugar level is less than 100 gm/dl (5.6 mmol/L). This can be tested during routine blood work or using a home glucometer test.

Human growth hormone, or HGH, is responsible for muscle growth and repair—for example, after injury or exercise. It helps build and maintain lean mass (muscle) and burn fat. It peaks during sleep and allows for the breakdown of stored glucose, so you have energy to start your day.

Cortisol is a hormone produced in the adrenal glands, which release cortisol based on our circadian rhythm. Cortisol can also be released in response to stress and low blood sugar levels. When the adrenal glands sense that blood sugar is getting too low, cortisol is released, creating new glucose and releasing it into the bloodstream. Cortisol works in opposition to insulin—cortisol raises blood sugar levels and insulin lowers them.

Cortisol, insulin, and HGH are in flux throughout a 24-hour period, mostly peaking in the morning and decreasing in the evening, which suggests morning is the best time for a meal. To improve your cardiovascular and metabolic health, eat to match the peak levels of these hormones.

What Happens When Insulin, Glucose, and Hormones Don't Work

Sometimes, your insulin, glucose, and hormones run into some problems. Here's a breakdown on what happens when each of these biological components don't work.

INSULIN

When you think of insulin issues, you may think of diabetes. Type 1 diabetes is a condition in which a person no longer makes insulin. Without insulin, their blood sugar will rise uncontrollably, which can have serious short- and long-term consequences. These individuals must take insulin every day. Before insulin was discovered, diabetes was a fatal disease. A person with type 2 diabetes can still make insulin, but doesn't make enough; the insulin they make doesn't work properly; or both. These individuals can take medications that help the pancreas produce more insulin, help the insulin meet up with the cell receptors, or both. Some require insulin injections as well. If you have insulin resistance, your insulin levels remain high, you store fat, develop more insulin resistance, and the cycle continues.

GLUCOSE

Excess glucose generally results from insulin resistance. It's dangerous to have blood glucose levels that are too high. People with diabetes who have chronic uncontrolled blood sugar are at significant risk for health issues, including vision loss, kidney failure, nerve damage, and blood vessel damage. When glucose levels are high, your body won't burn fat for fuel.

HGH

HGH deficiency in adults is linked to increased body fat, less muscle, decreased bone density, fatigue, lack of stamina, high blood fats, and a greater risk of diabetes and heart disease.

CORTISOL

In some conditions, the adrenal glands don't produce enough cortisol. When this occurs spontaneously, it is called Addison's disease. Low cortisol levels can also occur from cancer and infections and result in weakness, fatigue, and dizziness. You may also experience weight loss, lack of appetite, muscle aches, and other symptoms. Conversely, excess cortisol is called Cushing's syndrome, which causes weight gain.

How Fasting Helps

One key benefit of fasting is the metabolic switch ("the switch") in which the body changes from using glucose as the main fuel to using stored fat instead. The switch happens after about 12 hours of fasting and results in a decrease in blood sugar and insulin and a reduction in insulin resistance. When insulin goes down, the counter-regulatory hormone HGH goes up; HGH can help prevent the loss of bone and muscle.

Fasting also raises cortisol levels, as fasting is a stress to the body. You can manage this stress by choosing an appropriate fasting protocol, such as the ones discussed in this book, and coupling that with a regular stress management practice.

The Role of Autophagy

Autophagy (*auto* = self + *phagy* = *eating*) is the body's way of cleaning out damaged cells to create new, healthier ones in their place. It's described as a house-keeping function to eliminate damaged components that could otherwise become toxic. Autophagy occurs during fasting, and specifically during ketosis, after the body has used up stored glucose. Autophagy has been shown to play a major role in protecting against chronic conditions including diabetes, heart disease, cancer, and neurodegenerative diseases and may have anti-aging or rejuvenating effects, too.

Autophagy is also thought to be the reason for the anti-aging effects of calorie restriction. A Toronto-based physician using intermittent fasting for his obese patients credits autophagy for their lack of excess skin or the need for skin removal surgery despite significant weight loss. In addition, autophagy is credited with improving the appearance of intermittent fasters' skin.

FAQ: HOW INTERMITTENT FASTING WORKS

Q. If IF lowers blood sugar, will I have low blood sugar?

A. Unless you already suffer from low blood sugar (hypoglycemia), IF would not likely cause this problem. However, if you take medication to lower blood sugar, discuss proper medication adjustments with your diabetes educator.

Q. If I eat, will it break my fast?

A. Yes, eating or drinking anything other than water, unsweetened black coffee, or tea will break your fast.

Q. I don't have diabetes and my blood sugar is normal. Do I still need to lower them?

A. Your body has three different fuels it can use for energy: carbohydrates (glucose), fats (fatty acids), and proteins (amino acids). If your body has glucose, either as blood glucose or stored glucose, it will burn that first. You must use up the glucose before the body will break down fat stores, so yes, even with normal blood sugar levels, you want to lower them to tap into fat burning.

Q. *Aren't ketones a bad thing?*

A. Ketones are produced by the body as a by-product of using fat for energy. Although it's possible to have ketone levels that are too high—a condition called ketoacidosis—this is unlikely to occur in people who don't have type 1 diabetes (see more on page 18).

Q. *If I don't eat, won't my body use my muscles for fuel?*

A. No. After using glucose and glycogen for fuel, the body's next fuel source is fat. The body doesn't use muscle protein for fuel until you are at about 7 percent body fat.

Q. *I've heard that if you don't eat, your body slows its metabolism to compensate. Is this true?*

A. Intermittent fasting does not appear to lower the metabolic rate. In fact, IF seems to be protective of the metabolic rate in a way that continuous calorie restriction is not. IF definitely goes against some previously established ideas on this subject.

Is It Safe?

Safety is an important consideration when considering intermittent fasting. You'll need to consider your unique medical and health needs, as well as which method might be most appropriate for your specific situation and goals.

Most studies show no safety concerns with intermittent fasting, but these studies also exclude certain people from participating. This is why you should consult a medical expert if you have an underlying health issue and are considering IF. Exclusion criteria for these studies include shift workers, smokers, women who recently gave birth or who are breastfeeding, those taking medication, those with a history of cerebrovascular disease, hypertension, psychiatric conditions, cancer, and workers in high-risk occupations, such as crane operators, bus drivers, or pilots. If you are taking medication, consult with your doctor or pharmacist before fasting; if you are in a high-risk occupation, try fasting on your days off to see how your body reacts.

The duration of your intermittent-fasting program is also important to consider. A study of intermittent fasting may take place over 12 weeks and find no safety issue, but no long-term studies have been done. The longest follow-up I found was a one-year study with a two-year follow-up, where no significant weight loss was recorded as the participants didn't continue with fasting.

It's best to start gradually and pay attention to how you feel. If you can monitor your blood sugar, blood pressure, or other parameters, do so.

DO NOT DO THIS WHEN INTERMITTENT FASTING

Intermittent fasting should not be attempted if you have/are:

- A history of an eating disorder that is not well resolved
- An active eating disorder, such as anorexia, bulimia, or orthorexia
- Are a child who has not yet reached full adult height
- Breastfeeding
- Low blood sugar
- Pregnant
- Taking medication that requires food on a consistent schedule
- Uncontrolled diabetes
- Underweight or need to gain weight

Although not a complete contraindication, gout also calls for caution, as some research has shown elevated uric acid levels when intermittent fasting. Discuss with your physician whether more frequent uric acid testing is warranted.

Myths About Intermittent Fasting

You might be hesitant to try intermittent fasting because of something you read or heard. I'll dispel some common myths so you can decide what's best for you.

Fasting is dangerous. There are several ways to fast safely. When starting, consider and follow a protocol that's been researched and published.

Fasting puts your body into starvation mode. Biochemical changes take place during the fasting portion of your program. But because the fast is only temporary and followed by healthy eating, you're not starving. The body has an energy reserve of 161,000 calories. The energy needed for a 24-hour fast ranges from 1,600 to 6,000 calories (depending on activity level), so you have plenty of stored energy.

Breakfast is the most important meal of the day. This is kind of true. Several studies outline the benefits of breakfast, including healthy metabolic measurements, improved attention and cognitive function, a higher intake of vitamins and minerals, and prevention of weight gain. In addition, skipping breakfast may reduce physical activity and endurance exercise performance throughout the day. But just because a fasting protocol has you skip breakfast doesn't mean fasting can't be beneficial. We'll explore the benefits in chapter 2. Also, breakfast can be included in several protocols, so there's no need to limit yourself to a protocol that skips it if you want breakfast.

All the research is done on rats. Although there's a substantial amount of animal (mostly rat) research on intermittent fasting, there are also human studies that include individuals of normal weight, obese individuals, and people who have prediabetes and diabetes.

Intermittent fasting is hard. Some programs, like alternate-day fasting, have reported an increase in hunger, but not all protocols do. In fact, some report that hunger reduces on fasting days. If you're concerned about hunger, consider a conservative time-restricted feeding program.

You just eat more on nonfast days. Research shows this isn't true. In a study of people doing alternate-day fasting for eight weeks, the participants ate 95 to 100 percent of their calorie needs on their eating days and didn't overindulge.

I'm going to lose muscle when I fast. When you fast, your levels of growth hormone, responsible for maintaining muscle mass, increase. In a 12-week study of alternate-day fasting and/or exercise, participants maintained their muscle and lost fat.

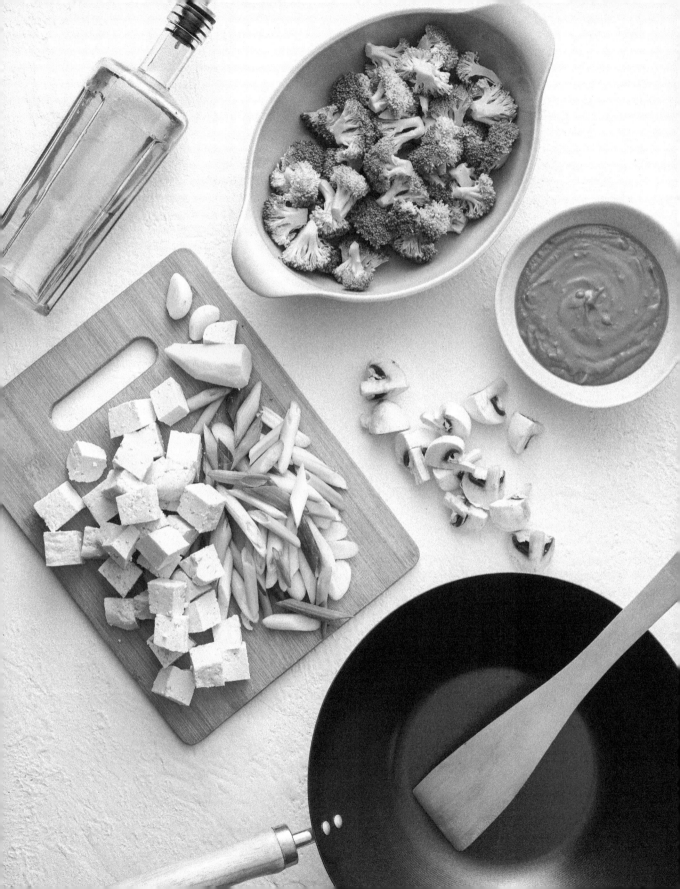

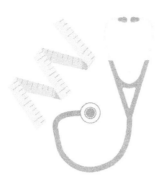

CHAPTER TWO

The Benefits of Intermittent Fasting

Weight loss is a popular benefit of intermittent fasting, but there are many other benefits. I describe them in this chapter, as well as the results from human research trials.

Weight Loss

For decades, the traditional approach to weight loss has been to eat a little bit less every day. This is called continuous calorie restriction. The difficulty with this method, as the name states, is that it's *continuous*. You need to count calories every day, measure food intake, or follow a meal plan.

For many, the possibility of a break from daily calorie restriction and eating a normal diet while still losing weight is appealing. This drives the interest in intermittent fasting. But which approach is better—continuous calorie restriction or IF?

A 2019 review pooled the results of 11 different studies comparing the two diet approaches. The results showed that the various intermittent-fasting regimens provided equivalent weight loss to continuous calorie restriction.

Three studies of time-restricted feeding were also analyzed: one using a 10- to 12-hour eating window, another using an eight-hour eating window, and the third in which participants ate breakfast 90 minutes later than usual and dinner 90 minutes earlier. The first two studies showed weight loss; the third showed fat loss without weight loss.

In essence these studies show that you can achieve weight loss through intermittent fasting without continuous calorie restriction.

Fat Loss

Intermittent fasting is most known for its weight-loss benefits. Studies confirm that there is fat loss on the regimens.

Some studies also specify that participants lose visceral fat through intermittent fasting and continuous calorie restriction. This type of fat is in the deeper abdominal layer and is responsible for creating inflammation in the body. Inflammation is linked to many chronic diseases, so losing this type of fat has benefits beyond just aesthetics.

Maintaining Muscle Mass

Research shows what happens when athletes combine IF and continue resistance training. Male athletes who ate within an eight-hour eating window lost more body fat compared to males who ate in a 12-hour eating window. Both groups, however, were able to maintain their muscle mass.

Diabetes Management and Insulin Control

Studies show tremendous benefits of intermittent fasting as it pertains to managing diabetes and insulin. One case study focused on men with type 2 diabetes on insulin who used an intermittent fasting schedule. Two men fasted every other day and one fasted three days a week. The improvement in their blood sugar was so dramatic that all were able to come off insulin between 5 and 18 days after beginning intermittent fasting. They also were able to reduce their oral diabetes medications. Two eventually came off all meds, and the third was able to reduce several medications. It's important to note that their insulin and medications were reduced in consultation with their doctor.

In a one-year study of people with type 2 diabetes, one group did a continuous calorie restriction diet and another group did 5:2 intermittent fasting (5 days eating normally and 2 days fasting; see chapter 3 for more on fasting protocols). At the conclusion of that year, most participants maintained some aspects of portion control or intermittent fasting. After two years, they were still able to maintain their lower dose of diabetes medication. However, those in the IF group were able to reduce their insulin more substantially than those in the continuous calorie restriction group. Weight and body fat loss was maintained, as was muscle mass.

A main diabetes measurement used in this study is called hemoglobin A1c (HgbA1c). In simple terms, think of it as a measure of your average blood sugar level over the past three months. The HgbA1c value was higher two years after the trial began; however, the researchers described that a natural rise in HgbA1c happens over time and it's been measured to be 0.3 percent per year—in this trial, it increased 0.3 percent in two years.

The overall conclusion is that intermittent fasting is as effective as continuous calorie restriction for people who have type 2 diabetes.

When you have diabetes and are interested in intermittent fasting, there are three main considerations: medication adjustment, frequency of blood sugar testing, and fluid intake. You'll need to adjust your diabetes medication on your fasting day. Since some diabetes medications are rapid onset and others are delayed, adjusting medication may not be as straightforward as simply reducing the dose on your fasting day.

I recommend working with your diabetes care team. If your team isn't familiar with IF, there's an excellent publication you can bring to your team that provides recommendations for adjusting diabetes medication while fasting. Check the chapter 2 reference section (page 177) for info on the paper by Grajower (2018).

Diabetes Medication

One risk of intermittent fasting when you have diabetes is hypoglycemia, or low blood sugar, particularly if you're taking insulin or sulfonylureas. Experiencing low blood sugar on other diabetes medication is rare but not unheard of.

Ketosis and Ketoacidosis

During your fast, your body may start producing ketones. When your body produces ketones, you're said to be in ketosis. This happens when the glycogen in the liver is used up, generally about 12 hours into your fast. In people with insulin resistance (typically, people with type 2 diabetes), the switch can take longer.

Ketosis is not the same as ketoacidosis, a dangerous side-effect of uncontrolled diabetes. Ketoacidosis occurs when there's a shortage of insulin and excess production of ketones to the point that the blood pH drops. It's more common in type 1 diabetes when a person is first diagnosed or when they are ill. Symptoms include extreme thirst and urination and high blood sugar. This requires immediate medical attention.

Disease Prevention

Research on disease prevention through intermittent fasting has focused on cardiovascular disease, diabetes, cancer, Alzheimer's, and rheumatoid arthritis. Here, I'll discuss IF's relationship to prevention of these diseases.

Preventing Diabetes

Several studies of intermittent fasting have shown improvement in insulin resistance. These results suggest that insulin resistance can be improved, implying that type 2 diabetes could be prevented.

One study concluded that every three-hour increase in nightly fasting was associated with an approximate 20 percent lower likelihood of having HbA1c at or above a prediabetes level. It also improved the blood sugar level. Researchers from the University of California took these results a step further by pointing out that high blood sugar and HgbA1c are also associated with breast cancer in women and suggested that lengthening the nighttime fast has potential to help prevent breast cancer as well.

Preventing Cardiovascular Disease

Members of The Church of Jesus Christ of Latter-day Saints in Utah have lower rates of coronary artery disease than the rest of the country. Church teachings include a monthly fast for 24 hours. A report from the University of Utah determined that the fasting was associated with a lower risk of coronary heart disease. This was true even when the researchers accounted for the members' avoidance of smoking, alcohol, and caffeine.

The protection of metabolic health was also seen in a study of overweight adults who were asked to limit their eating window from 8:00 a.m. until 2:00 p.m. Researchers also noted anti-aging effects of time-restricted feeding.

Improved Blood Lipids

What do the studies of intermittent fasting say about blood lipids, blood pressure, and inflammation? Trials show that intermittent fasting improves blood lipid levels, raising the HDL and lowering the LDL, total cholesterol, and triglycerides.

Improvements in blood lipids with intermittent fasting can occur even if weight loss doesn't. Blood lipid levels have also improved with either a high-fat/low-carb diet or a low-fat/high-carb diet when part of an IF protocol. Research shows that if you combine intermittent fasting with exercise you can improve these results even more.

Improved Blood Pressure

Studies of time-restricted feeding have shown improved blood pressure, insulin levels, and insulin sensitivity when participants ate early or in the middle of the day. Their metabolic health was either not affected or worsened when they ate late in the day. Other studies, including a study of 5:2 (see page 31) and two alternate-day fasting studies, found improved blood pressure.

These are important considerations if you have high blood pressure and are considering which time-restricted feeding protocol is best for you. Ideally, you can monitor your blood pressure to make sure you're getting the desired results.

Reduced Inflammation

Short-term inflammation helps you heal; conversely, long-term (chronic) inflammation is very damaging, creating an environment that allows cancer, heart disease, Alzheimer's disease, and other conditions to take hold.

A 2015 study compared the length of an overnight fast to the blood levels of inflammation and insulin resistance. Each 10 percent increase in the proportion of calories consumed in the evening was associated with a 3 percent rise in inflammation. Another finding associated longer nighttime fasting with reduced inflammation when women ate less than 30 percent of their total calories in the evening. Researchers also found that eating one additional snack or meal during the day was associated with reduced inflammation.

Improved Sleep

In one study, people who followed a 10- to 12-hour eating window of time-restricted feeding for 16 weeks reported improved sleep, which continued for a year, until the study's conclusion.

Living Longer

As we age, the genes that regulate our internal clocks become disorganized and disrupted. The disruption in our circadian clock is associated with a variety of chronic diseases, including heart disease, ulcers, diabetes, and cancer.

Lifestyle choices can also contribute to this decline. For example, erratic eating and sleeping routines, shift work, or jet lag can contribute to a dysfunctional internal clock, leading to unhealthy levels in hormones, metabolism, and more. These unhealthy levels are linked to the same chronic diseases associated with aging. In essence, your lifestyle choices may accelerate—or slow—the aging process.

In addition, your body's cells respond to repeated fasting with an adaptive stress response that leads to greater antioxidant defenses and DNA repair. These adaptive responses are credited with the increase in longevity seen in animal models.

Reduced Cancer Risk and an Adjunct to Cancer Treatment

Most IF research has focused on the metabolic changes that occur with intermittent fasting, such as reduced glucose, insulin resistance, and inflammation and how that could reduce the risk of cancer development. Some evidence shows that fasting can protect the body from the toxicity of chemotherapy and radiation while enhancing their effectiveness.

If you have cancer and are considering IF, discuss it with your oncologist. The benefits must be balanced with the risks, including the potential of unwanted weight loss, weakness, or loss of muscle, further compromising the immune system, or slowing wound healing at a vulnerable time.

Rheumatoid Arthritis

A review on IF for those with rheumatoid arthritis combined the results of 31 studies and concluded that a period of fasting followed by a vegetarian diet helped improve pain, stiffness, and inflammation.

Increased Energy Levels

In one study, healthy people with an erratic eating schedule restricted their eating to a 10- to 12-hour window for 16 weeks. They lost weight and felt more energetic. In fact, they felt so good, they continued with the eating plan even after the study was finished.

Improved Asthma Symptoms

Adults with asthma who followed alternate-day fasting for two months found improvement in their asthma symptoms and experienced weight loss and reduced inflammation.

PCOS

Specific female reproductive conditions, such as polycystic ovarian syndrome (PCOS), pregnancy, and menopause, can affect a woman's insulin function. Although more research is needed, a study of women with PCOS during Ramadan fasting shows a reduction in stress hormone levels. It is hypothesized that intermittent fasting can help with PCOS.

FAQ: INTERMITTENT FASTING BENEFITS

Q. Will I lose weight right away?

A. You'll probably lose weight more dramatically after your fast day(s). If your weight loss is consistent with research, you'll lose about the same as you would on a more traditional low-calorie diet.

Q. Do I have to give up my favorite foods?

A. As long as you follow your eating and fasting protocol, you don't need to give up your favorite foods (within reason, of course!).

Q. Do I have to count calories?

A. You don't need to count calories on your eating days—simply eat a healthy balanced diet within reason. But if you follow a modified fast that allows some intake on the fasting day (usually 500 to 750 calories), you'll need to plan these calories.

Q. *Will I overeat on my eating day and cancel out my fast day?*

A. Research says you won't. Most people can eat a reasonable amount of food after fasting. It helps to stay hydrated and practice mindful eating—sit, eat slowly, focus on your senses, and stop when you feel satisfied.

Q. *Besides weight loss and health, what other benefits are there?*

A. You might find fasting a real productivity hack, as on your fasting day, you'll spend less time doing meal prep and eating.

Q. *Will I be able to concentrate when fasting?*

A. Many people report feeling very clear-headed during intermittent fasting.

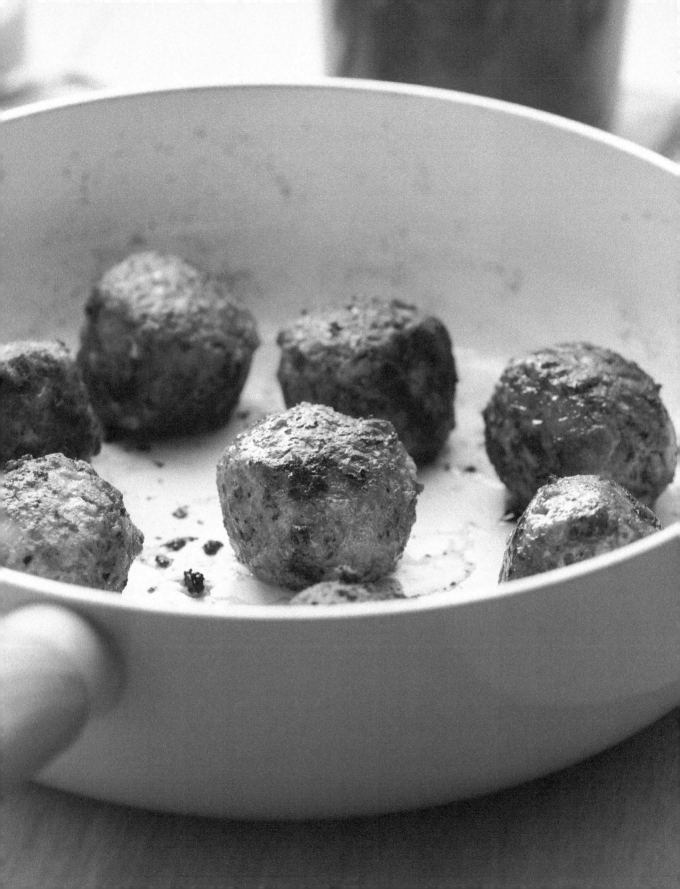

CHAPTER THREE

Feeding and Fasting Windows

There are a variety of ways to implement intermittent fasting, and the nice thing about it is, you can choose the one that appeals to you. You can even try more than one way and settle into the program that best aligns with your lifestyle and routine.

Daily Fasting Methods

Daily fasting methods, also called time-restricted feeding, are done every day. This gets your body into a routine and syncs your peripheral clocks with your master clock. These methods divide the 24-hour day into a fasting window and a feeding window.

When choosing the times for your feeding and fasting windows, consistency is key, so pick something you can stick with on most days, including weekends.

12:12

For this method, you eat during a 12-hour window and fast for 12 hours (for example, an eating window from 9:00 a.m. to 9:00 p.m.). 12:12 is the easiest of the daily fasts and is ideal if you're new to intermittent fasting or if your current eating routine is erratic. Do not expect to lose very much weight on this plan. This plan is about achieving balance between time spent eating and not eating.

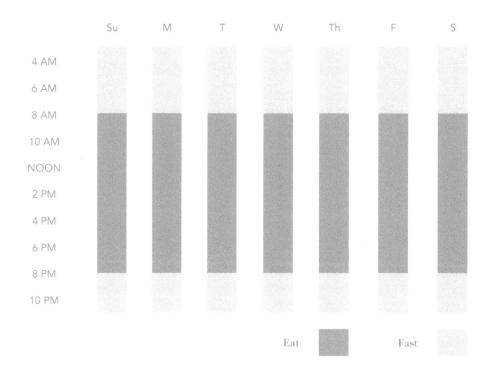

16:8 ("Leangains")

This is an intermediate fasting plan. You can build up to this from 12:12 by gradually shortening the eating window from 12 hours to 8. You should lose weight or fat on this plan, as you will be burning fatty acids for fuel toward the end of your fasting window. You will also get a decent amount of time in cellular-repair mode each day. In this method, you eat during an eight-hour window and fast for 16 hours. A book called *The Leangains Method* is based on 16:8 and is designed for sport and strength trainers who want to get as lean as possible while gaining strength.

To use this fasting method, choose your eight-hour eating window (for example, 9:00 a.m. until 5:00 pm or 12:00 p.m. until 8:00 p.m.). Studies indicate that keeping your eating window in the early or middle part of the day is better for weight loss, insulin levels, insulin sensitivity, and blood pressure. Many hormones and plasma lipids peak in the morning and drop in the evening, further suggesting the morning as optimal for food intake. But, ultimately, choose a schedule that works for you.

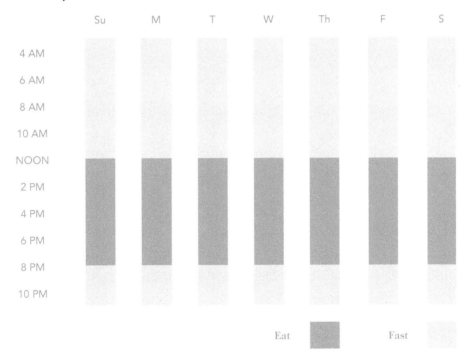

20:4 ("Warrior Diet")

On this program, you fast for 20 hours and eat during a four-hour window. Although, technically, this could be any four hours you choose, there is a specific 20:4 protocol called the Warrior Diet, named after a book of the same title.

Because you eat only during a four-hour window—and this is likely only one or two meals—you'll need to choose highly nutritious foods and get all your vitamins and minerals with them. This includes foods from all food groups and whole, not processed, foods. This protocol may appeal to you if you're busy during the day and often find you don't have time to eat.

In a 2007 study, normal-weight middle-aged people consumed all their calories for weight maintenance in either a four-hour window or three meals per day for six weeks. Over 25 percent of participants withdrew from the study, possibly due to hunger. Researchers found mixed results in blood lipids—some got worse (LDL and total cholesterol) and some got better (HDL and triglycerides). Interestingly, they lost body weight and fat despite the fact that calorie intake was not designed for weight loss in this study.

If you choose this plan, monitor your weight, blood lipids, and blood pressure.

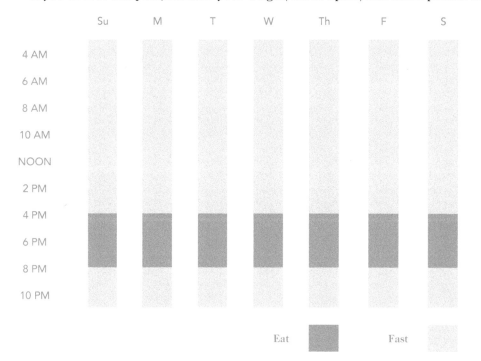

One Meal a Day ("OMAD")

This is an advanced fasting plan, so don't choose this routine if this is your very first time fasting. Eating one meal a day, or OMAD, is even more restrictive as it's considered a 23:1 (fasting 23 hours, eating 1 hour). You can build up to this from 16:8 by gradually shortening the eating window from eight hours to one. But, as an evidence-based health professional, I have a hard time recommending 23:1.

How is it possible to meet your requirements for vitamins, minerals, fiber, and protein in one meal? Why be so strict when other less-stringent programs offer results? There's no published research supporting the efficacy of 23:1. There was one study that tested "one meal a day versus three meals per day," but participants had four hours to eat.

I don't recommend starting with this program; instead, choose another method first, like 16:8 (see page 27), 5:2 (see page 31), or alternate-day fasting (see page 31), which have been studied in the short term and found to be safe.

I should mention that the term "OMAD" is rather fuzzy in the fasting community. Although by definition it is 23:1, many people use the term to simply mean they eat one meal a day, but don't restrict themselves to a one-hour window. In that way, it's more like a 20:4 but can include "one meal" spread out over four hours.

Weekly Fasting Methods

Where the previous section looked at dividing your 24-hour day into eating and fasting windows, the protocols in this section divide the week into eating and fasting days. Let's explore.

24 Hour ("Eat, Stop, Eat")

This protocol and the book by the same name were written by Brad Pilon. He recommends fasting once or twice a week for 24 hours. For the remainder of the week, make sensible choices.

To do this, decide on your 24-hour window. For example, eat lunch at noon then take only low-calorie fluids for dinner. Skip breakfast the next morning and eat lunch at noon. It offers a lot of flexibility, and you never need to go an entire day without food.

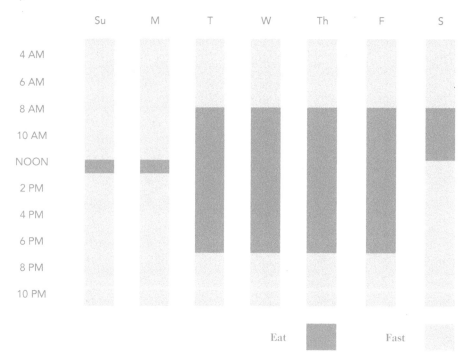

5:2

5:2 is a great starting point if you're completely new to fasting and want to lose weight while not having to fast every day. The 5:2 protocol recommends 5 days of eating normally and 2 days of fasting, usually consecutive but not always. This protocol is not a water fast. You restrict your intake to about 25 percent of your needs, called *a modified fast*. Typically, you'll consume 500 to 750 calories on fasting days. The other five days you'll eat your usual diet, within reason.

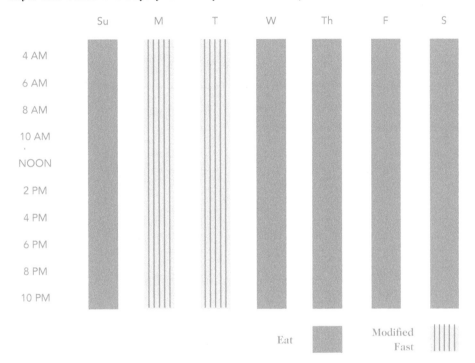

Alternate-Day Fasting

This program was described by Dr. Krista Varady, assistant professor and author of *The Every Other Day Diet*. For this, you don't water fast, but instead do a modified fast with 500 calories. Out of all the intermittent fasts covered in this book, this is the plan that gives you the longest stretch of time continuously fasting. You may imagine you get a 24-hour fast every other day, but it's longer than that, as you count the hours from your dinner the previous night to breakfast on the day after your fast.

You can think of this as a 36:12, alternating one day of fasting with one day of eating normally. In this program, you'd eat at your normal times (for example, 7:00 a.m., 1:00 p.m., and 7:00 p.m.) one day, then consume 500 calories the next day, then resume eating on the third day at 7:00 a.m., having done a modified fast for 36 hours. Some choose a water fast on their fast days and skip the 500 calories.

This differs from the 24-hour "eat, stop, eat" method in that the fast is longer and happens every other day, not just twice a week. Think of it as the next step up from 24-hour fasting. With this long stretch of fasting comes the benefits associated with using ketones as your main source of fuel and activating repair mode longer.

I would suggest using the modified fast version first or working up to this by trying some of the other fasting methods first. You can progress to this protocol if you aren't experiencing any side effects.

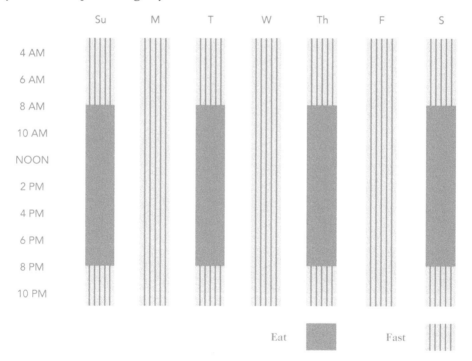

HOW EXERCISE CAN FIT INTO
YOUR FASTING WINDOW

To get the most out of your workouts, plan high-intensity workouts and weight training on days/times when you're eating so you can fuel up after working out. Experiment with exercising during fasting times to see if you still get a good workout. During fasting days/times, it makes sense to maximize fat burn by doing aerobic, fat-burning workouts. You'll want to give your body time to adapt to the effects of fasting—and don't start fasting right before a big race or competition. Instead start fasting in your training window to give yourself time to adapt and monitor your speed, endurance, and strength so you can make appropriate adjustments to your IF and exercise schedule.

Extended Fasting Methods

This type of fasting is more advanced than daily (time-restricted feeding) or weekly (24 hour, 5:2, and 36:12). This should not be the first fast you try. In fact, if you find a method of fasting that's comfortable for you and helps you achieve your goals, don't feel like you need to progress to extended fasts.

48-Hour Fasts

In a 48-hour fast, you begin after dinner on day one, then fast all of day two, then resume eating with dinner on day three. You could do this for any meal, if you break the fast at the same meal on day three. You can choose to do this as a modified fast by consuming about 500 calories a day, or you can choose to consume only water, unsweetened black coffee, or tea.

This protocol is only expected to be followed once or twice a month, not every week, and it is not for beginners—you may also want to try a modified-fast version before moving to water only.

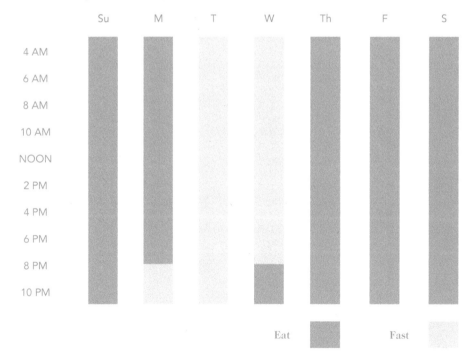

48 Hour + Fasts

Long-term fasting is three days or more and keeps you in ketosis longer. Ketosis has many benefits for metabolism including increasing stress resistance, breakdown of fat stores, and autophagy (see page 18).

Ideally, these fasts should be done in consultation with your physician. Use caution if you're taking medications, especially if they need to be taken with food. Your ghrelin (hunger hormone) levels will peak on day two, so if you can get past that, the hunger reduces and doesn't keep increasing.

While some people may start their days very early, we based the following chart on a day that begins at 8:00 a.m. and eating that ends at 8:00 p.m. Even on the days you're not fasting, eating late at night is not recommended. Ideally, you want to keep your eating window on non-fasting days to 12 hours.

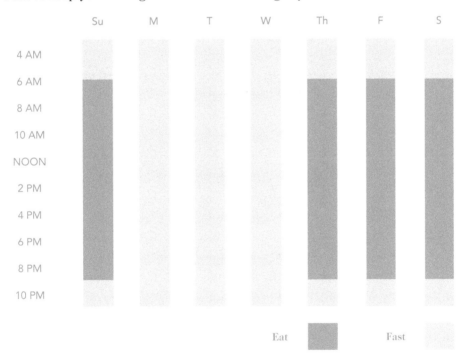

Let's explore some of the popular questions about feeding and fasting windows.

Q. *Is a morning or evening feeding schedule better?*

A. When you do time-restricted feeding you have two options for timing: to extend your overnight fast into morning by skipping or delaying breakfast, or to eat an early dinner and begin your fast in the evening, which extends into overnight. Health research supports the first option, but the second option is more popular among fasters. Keep reading to find out about matching your eating with your chronotype (whether you're an early bird or night owl).

Bottom line: Choose a schedule you can stick to on most days and monitor your results.

Q. *How many times a day should I eat?*

A. There doesn't seem to be agreement on this. Studies have shown that eating often is healthier for cholesterol, cardiovascular health, healthy weight, and blood sugar. A study from the University of Alabama suggests that meals less than four hours apart may improve fluctuations in blood sugar. Other studies have shown the opposite—that eating only one or two meals a day is better to lower body weight and reduce diabetes risk.

A 2019 review suggests the combination of the timing of your meals, the frequency of meals, and the length of your overnight fast are probably most important. In essence, a long overnight fast and regular meal timing are important no matter how many meals you eat on a regular basis.

Q. *Does it matter if I eat at the same time every day?*

A. A regular eating schedule allows the peripheral clocks to be in sync with the master clock. It was also pointed out in one study that shift workers, transcontinental travelers, and people with irregular work schedules often have irregular bowel habits including constipation and diarrhea. If this is an issue for you, keep yourself on a regular schedule with your chosen IF regimen.

Q. *What if I don't feel like eating in the morning?*

A. We have genes that determine our internal clocks. Some of us are early birds and some of us are night owls—that is your chronotype. In a study of weight-loss diets, participants achieved more weight loss when the calorie distribution matched their chronotype (early birds eating a larger meal earlier/night owls eating a larger meal later). Most research seems to indicate that having the larger meal in the earlier part of the day is better, but this can be difficult to fit into our lifestyle and difficult to stomach if you're just not a morning person.

This research was not done on IF, so it's uncertain how these two elements fit together, but I recommend considering your chronotype to decide when to have your big meal of the day. See the Resources section (see page 171) for a link to an online test to determine your chronotype.

PART TWO

How to Apply Intermittent Fasting to Your Life

Now that you understand the types of intermittent fasting and their benefits and risks, it's time to get practical with how-to information. In the following chapters, we'll explore the many feeding and fasting windows and how to choose the right one for you. Then, I offer some final advice so you can get started!

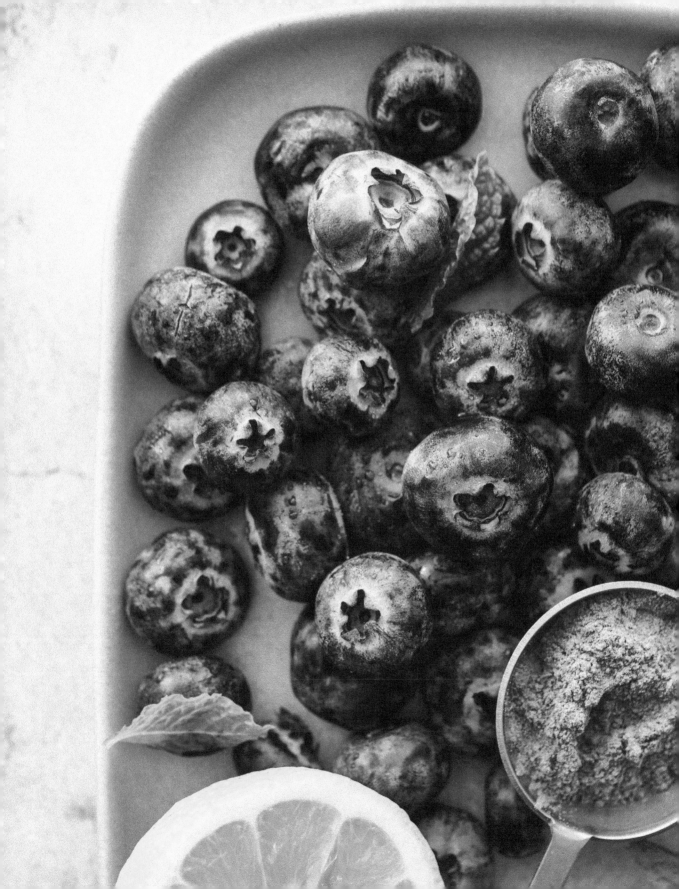

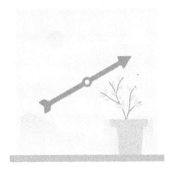

CHAPTER FOUR

How to Choose the Right Feeding and Fasting Window for You

In the following sections, we'll focus on your specific needs and how to best accommodate them. More than one feeding/fasting window may be right for you and may require some trial and error, so keep this in mind.

Consider Why You're Fasting

Although research shows IF can help with weight loss, blood sugar control, and reduced cardiovascular risk, no research has done a head-to-head comparison of which IF method is best. Let's dive into some things to consider about your options.

If You Want to Lose Weight

The following methods have at least one human clinical trial showing that fasting leads to weight loss. These methods are listed in order of difficulty, from easy (12:12, 5:2) to more difficult (20:4, alternate-day fasting):

▸ Daily fasting methods:

→ 12:12

→ 16:8

→ 20:4

▸ Weekly fasting methods:

→ 5:2

→ Alternate-day fasting

One Meal a Day (OMAD) 23:1 has limited research. The 24-hour ("Eat, Stop, Eat") method lacks published research. Extended-fasting methods should be done under medical supervision and are not recommended as your first exposure to IF.

If You're Managing Insulin

The only clinical trials conducted including people with type 2 diabetes involved 5:2 weekly fasting schedules. One case study describes men with type 2 diabetes who did 24-hour fasts three times per week with good results.

When taking insulin, the bigger concern is not which IF protocol you follow, but whether you have a diabetes educator who can help you manage your diabetes. Keep a fast-acting source of glucose on hand in case you need to treat low blood sugar and reduce long-acting insulin for fasting days. *If you experience low blood sugar, treat it even though it will break your fast.*

If You Want General Wellness

This is straightforward: Choose the method that appeals to you and is the best fit for your lifestyle. If you're uncertain, consult your physician and/or a dietitian for guidance.

Consider Your Lifestyle

To be successful with intermittent fasting and achieving your goals, the program needs to fit with your lifestyle. Here are some considerations to keep in mind.

If You Work A Standard Eight-Hour Workday

Having a regular routine, at least with work hours, makes intermittent fasting easier. You can choose to either shorten your eating window or choose one of the weekly fasting methods.

Some standard protocols that work well with an eight-hour workday include:

→ 5:2
→ 12:12
→ 14:10
→ 16:8
→ 18:6

It's also important to consider:

► How hungry are you during the day? When are you most hungry?

  → Choose a feeding window that allows you to eat when you're most hungry. If hungrier during midday, adopt a time-restricted eating window that includes a big lunch around noon or 1:00 p.m. and finish eating for the day by about 6:00 p.m.

► Do you need to eat first thing in the morning?

  → If the answer is no, push back your first meal of the day in your time-restricted window.
  → If yes, plan your eating window to include breakfast and an early dinner or late lunch.

- Do you skip breakfast at home and eat something when you get to work?

  → This is ideal for 16:8, or possibly 20:4, in which you delay breakfast.

- How busy are you at work?

  → If you're busy, you may prefer to focus on work and eat when you get home.

- Are there some days when you're busier and find it hard to stop to eat?

  → If so, try 5:2 and limit your eating on those busy days, but stay hydrated.

- When do you work out?

  → You can do low-intensity workouts on a fasting day, but for higher-intensity activities, eat after the workout to properly fuel your muscles.

- Do you eat with the other people in your household? Do you have a work dinner or happy hour? When?

  → Plan your eating window so you can eat with others, especially if there are routine after-hours events to keep in mind.

- Do you have evening commitments that involve food or activity that need to be considered?

  → Push back your first meal of the day to accommodate this, or fast the next day.

Just because the time-restricted feeding has standard protocols, there is nothing stopping you from doing something unique to you, like 15:9, 17:7, or 19:5, or having a range of fasting windows depending on your schedule; for example, 15:9 on most days and 18:6 on days when you have a commitment after work.

If You Travel a Lot

You might travel often and may even cross time zones but still want to participate in intermittent fasting. Here are things to consider about IF and travel.

▶ How long is your trip?

→ For longer stays, adjust to local time. If so, you can fast on the plane and break your fast in your host country with a meal that corresponds to local time.

→ For quick trips, fast through the local mealtimes and stick with your home eating schedule. This may also help reduce jet lag upon returning home.

▶ If your normal eating time is in the middle of the night while traveling, you may prefer to sleep through it and extend your fast.

▶ Do you find eating while traveling inconvenient?

→ If so, consider fasting right through your travel day—just stay hydrated.

▶ How hungry are you when you travel?

→ Sometimes travel itself can affect your appetite. Listen to your body—if you aren't hungry, extend your fast.

→ If you are hungrier, remember that even 12:12 is a form of fasting.

▶ Does air travel make you constipated? Fasting could make that worse. Stay hydrated, and if you eat, choose easily digested foods such as chicken, eggs, fish, nuts, oatmeal, rice, toast, or yogurt.

▶ Does travel make you nauseous? If so, having something in your stomach may help.

▶ Do you take short trips often? If so, you might choose a 5:2 or 4:3 method in which your travel days are your fasting days, or vice versa.

▶ Do you like to try new foods?

→ You may prefer to eat three meals a day in your host country to take advantage of the cuisine, then fast when you return home, such as a 5:2 or 4:3 approach.

- How much control do you have over your eating schedule? Are you expected to attend work or social functions that involve eating with others?
  - → Try to get your agenda ahead of time so you can plan your fasts.
  - → You may need to participate in the functions and get back to fasting upon returning home.

There are no strict rules—listen to your body and go with it!

Traveling across time zones causes jet lag and upsets your circadian rhythm—it's just the way it is. Choosing to eat when it's light and fast when it's dark can help realign your master clock with your peripheral clocks. For this reason, a form of time-restricted feeding may make the most sense for travelers, but it's not the only option.

If You Have an Unpredictable Schedule

It's ideal to regulate your schedule as much as possible. If you can regulate it enough to follow time-restricted feeding, do so. Aim for a conservative 12:12 intermittent fasting schedule to start.

The next-best option would be alternate-day fasting, a 24-hour fast, or 5:2. But make sure your schedule isn't so unpredictable that you can't plan for healthy meals when you need to eat.

Intermittent fasting would be particularly challenging for occupations that are physically demanding on short notice, such as a firefighter, on-call performer, or per diem nurse. You can design your own unique schedule, even by combining two or more methods. For example, you may want to do 16:8 most days and a 36-hour fast once a month, if that works best. You can also fast one day a week or one day a month.

If You Have Kids or Are Very Social

You'll want to plan so you don't feel left out of important celebrations and milestones. You may prefer a fasting method in which you get to eat at least one meal a day.

Fasting methods that tend to be more social include protocols such as 16:8, in which you skip breakfast, but still enjoy lunch and dinner. If you're eating out, remember that if you have a reservation, you probably won't start eating until about 45 minutes after that time. So, consider what time you will open and close your eating window to include an evening out.

Most fasting schedules will accommodate family and social life, but you may need different fasts for different days. For example, you might do 20:4 Monday to Friday and 12:12 on the weekends. If you are doing 5:2 or 4:3, then, perhaps, you'll choose your fasting days during the week and save eating days for the weekend.

How to Get Started

There are three basic steps to prepare for fasting:

1. Figure out what you want. Get clear about your goal(s). Are they healthy? Do they lead to overall wellness? If yes, then proceed; if you're not sure, reconsider your needs.

2. Choose your feeding and fasting windows. There are many choices, so consider which is best for you.

3. Decide what to eat. Get inspiration from the recipes in this book.

Mental Preparation

Check in with yourself and be honest about your reasons for doing IF. They should be positive, healthy reasons that make you look forward to a healthy change, especially as you may encounter some challenges in the beginning, including hunger, cravings, and/or headaches. Be honest about your relationship with food, and if you feel that intermittent fasting may trigger disordered eating, please seek the help of a registered dietitian. With professional support, you can choose a healthy strategy to reach your goal that won't trigger a relapse or new eating disorder.

Physical Preparation

Here are ways to help you prepare:

- Don't start intermittent fasting before a major work project or a big race.
- Eat as you normally would the day before you start the fast.

- Remember, you've probably fasted before for a blood test or medical procedure and you got through it.
- Stay well hydrated and well rested.

Kitchen Preparation

A thoughtfully stocked kitchen will help you be successful while fasting. You'll need to stock up on healthy foods to eat during feeding days, as well as include plenty of options for modified-fast days, if that's the plan you choose. Get rid of tempting foods but remember, there isn't a "fasting diet." In theory, you should be able to eat your usual foods—just with more focus on *when* you eat them. Of course, you'll want portions to be reasonable—for example, it won't benefit you to eat twice as much during your feeding windows.

Family Preparation

Are you responsible for cooking for others? Will you be expected to continue this while you are fasting? It's important to talk with your family about how they can support you in achieving your goals. If you'll be cooking for others while you fast, consider preparing meals that aren't your favorites or preparing meals ahead of time. Organize food for your family in a way that makes it as easy as possible for you.

Avoiding Temptation

Don't make fasting harder than it has to be. If you have food items in your house that will tempt you, give them away or put them out of sight. Also, think about temptations outside of the home. Some creative ways to avoid those pitfalls include:

- Don't walk or drive by tempting shops or restaurants if there's another route you can take.
- Don't shop hungry—for anything, not just groceries. Tempting food is everywhere!
- Drink water, tea, or black coffee to help stave off hunger while fasting.

- If you want to go for a walk but don't trust yourself, leave your money at home.
- Keep busy. Time flies when you're mentally preoccupied.
- Remind yourself that you get to eat regular meals when it's time.

Going Shopping

Be proactive about what you're going to eat so you're not tempted to overdo it when your eating window opens. Make a list and shop on a feeding day after eating—not on a fasting day when you're hungry. One key to success is to keep foods on hand that you *want* to eat, and *not* keeping foods around that you *don't* want to eat. This can be a challenge if you live with other people who aren't on the same page. Be clear about what you need from them to help you succeed.

If you have health concerns and are following a specific diet, learn what you can eat by consulting with your doctor or a dietitian. If you're at risk for low blood sugar, have some dextrose tabs or other fast-absorbing carbs on hand for emergencies. Make sure you have enough glucose testing strips if you're monitoring diabetes. If you want to check for ketones, get some urine ketone testing strips. And have your favorite headache remedy on hand, just in case.

If you have diabetes, continue to follow the recommendations for a diabetic diet on your feeding day; namely limiting refined carbs, spacing out fruit servings, choosing whole grains (if including grains), and choosing healthy lean proteins and healthy fats.

EASING IN VERSUS JUMPING IN

Whether you ease in or jump in to IF is up to you, but easing in will help minimize side effects. If you're doing time-restricted feeding, this means gradually closing your eating window and expanding your fasting window. You can start with 12:12 and extend your fast in half-hour to one-hour increments at one end or both ends of your eating window.

To ease into a weekly fast, gradually restrict your intake on your fast day before going to a full fast. If you plan to do water only on your fast day, try a 500- to 750-calorie modified fast first. Much of this comes down to personality and preference. If you're prone to headaches, low blood pressure, or the hangries, ease into fasting.

What to Expect in the Beginning

Some things you may experience as you get started include:

- ▶ Bad breath
- ▶ Constipation
- ▶ Decreased energy
- ▶ Feeling cold
- ▶ Mood swings or bad temper
- ▶ Preoccupation with food

Let's look at how to manage three of the more common side effects.

Hunger Pangs

Drinking water, tea, or coffee can help ease hunger. Thankfully, the hunger won't last too long, so distracting yourself can also help. Remind yourself of your goals. I find it helps to tell myself that the hunger pang is the body asking for food, and when I don't feed it, my body will use my fat stores instead. If you must eat something, don't beat yourself up. You may be able to adjust for that by closing your eating window earlier or reducing what you eat.

Overeating

Until you hit your stride, you may find yourself overeating. Although many sources promise you can eat whatever you want as long as it's within your eating window, good judgment is also important. Eat what you would normally eat as a serving size. The savings in calories come from the meals or the days you skip eating, and you don't want to undo your good work.

Headaches

For many of us, headaches start with some warning signs. Keep yourself well hydrated, and if you feel a headache coming on, caffeine might help, so drink a black coffee or tea. You might invest in a topical headache remedy and keep your headache meds of choice on hand, especially if you're prone to migraines.

What Not to Expect

The following are some indications that your IF regimen is causing unhealthy consequences for you and that you need to scale back or stop fasting:

- Anxiety and/or depression
- Avoidance of your normal social circle and isolation at home
- Binge-eating behaviors
- Difficulty concentrating to the point that driving or another high-risk activity is impaired
- Disturbed sleep
- Fainting
- Feeling overly harsh or judgmental toward yourself
- Loss of menstrual cycle
- Inability to complete daily living activities
- Inability to function normally
- Rapid ongoing weight loss of more than 2 pounds per week

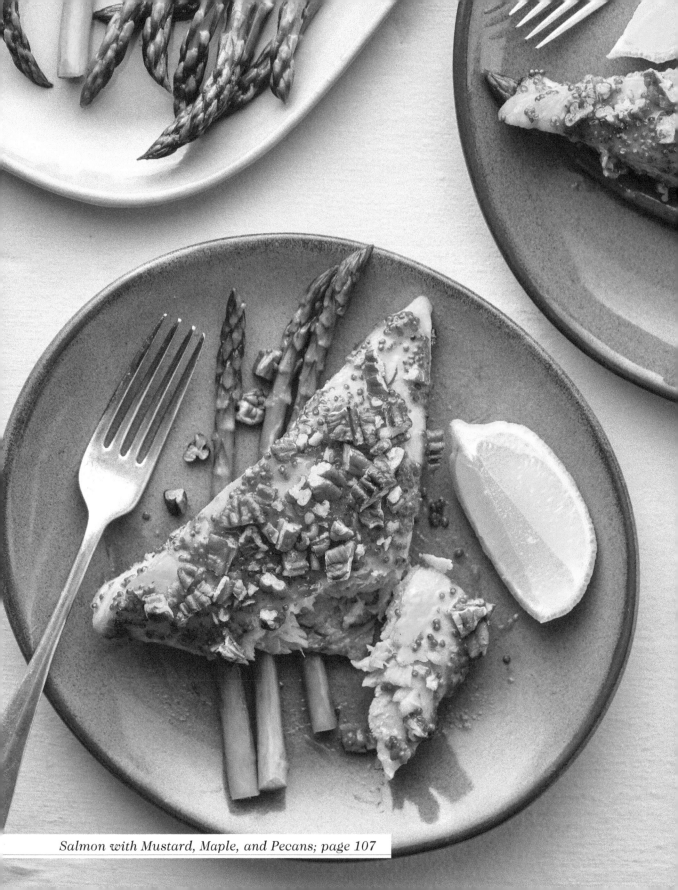

Salmon with Mustard, Maple, and Pecans; page 107

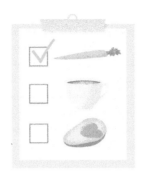

CHAPTER FIVE

Meal Plans for Fasting

This section presents meal plans for the various fasting and feeding schedules to give you an idea of what your week could look like. These will look different from diet meal plans, in that I'll focus on *when* (and in the case of modified fasts, how many calories) you should eat. Each meal plan will be accompanied by a sample meal plan of what to eat.

The 16:8 Meal Plan

For this plan, you'll have an eight-hour eating window and a 16-hour fasting window. Some evidence shows that keeping your eating window to daylight hours can help realign your master clock with your peripheral clocks and eating the bulk of your calories during the morning and midday is better than end of day. But ultimately, choose a plan that works best for you. For this sample chart, I chose times I thought would be most popular.

Sample Meal Plan

Breakfast: Sour Cream and Onion Egg Salad Lettuce Wraps (page 102)

Lunch: Lemony Chicken Soup with the soup variation of the broth (page 84)

Dinner: Crispy Baked Tofu, Broccoli, and Mushroom Stir-Fry with Peanut Sauce (page 134)

Sunday

Breakfast: 11:00 a.m.

Lunch: 3:00 p.m. (optional)

Dinner: finish by 7:00 p.m.

Monday

Breakfast: 11:00 a.m.

Lunch: 3:00 p.m. (optional)

Dinner: finish by 7:00 p.m.

Tuesday

Breakfast: 11:00 a.m.

Lunch: 3:00 p.m. (optional)

Dinner: finish by 7:00 p.m.

Wednesday

Breakfast: 11:00 a.m.

Lunch: 3:00 p.m. (optional)

Dinner: finish by 7:00 p.m.

Thursday

Breakfast: 11:00 a.m.

Lunch: 3:00 p.m. (optional)

Dinner: finish by 7:00 p.m.

Friday

Breakfast: 11:00 a.m.

Lunch: 3:00 p.m. (optional)

Dinner: finish by 7:00 p.m.

Saturday

Breakfast: 11:00 a.m.

Lunch: 3:00 p.m. (optional)

Dinner: finish by 7:00 p.m.

During the day, consume water to stay hydrated (see clean and dirty fasting, page 62).

The 5:2 Fast Meal Plan

The 5:2 plan is not a water-only fast; it's a modified fast. Your calorie intake for fasting days should be about 25 percent of your usual intake—500 to 750 calories for most people.

The big question is whether your two fasting days should be consecutive. Some people claim the second consecutive day of fasting is easier as your body gets used to it; others claim it's harder. Trial and error can help you determine what works for you. The research has used both methods.

This meal plan was designed with nonconsecutive fasting days, but customize it as you prefer. You can choose how many meals to distribute the 500 to 750 calories between; in this example, I use 3 meals, so it's about 150 to 250 calories per meal. If, however, taking three small meals makes you hungrier or makes it harder to stop eating, try one 500-calorie meal instead.

Modified Fasting Day Sample Meal Plan

Breakfast: Herbed Turkey Broth, 159 calories (page 86)

Lunch: Greek Village Salad, 207 calories (page 101)

Dinner: Vegetarian Chili with Cranberries, 138 calories (page 143)

Total Calories: 504

Eating Day Sample Meal Plan

Breakfast: Almond Smoothie with Dates and Cinnamon (page 94)

Lunch: Arugula Salad with Tuna (page 100)

Dinner: Lentil and Sweet Potato Tacos with Fresh Guacamole and Pico de Gallo (page 139)

Sunday

Breakfast: low-calorie meal

Lunch: low-calorie meal

Dinner: low-calorie meal

Monday

Breakfast: regular meal

Lunch: regular meal

Dinner: regular meal

Tuesday

Breakfast: regular meal

Lunch: regular meal

Dinner: regular meal

Wednesday

Breakfast: low-calorie meal

Lunch: low-calorie meal

Dinner: low-calorie meal

Thursday

Breakfast: regular meal

Lunch: regular meal

Dinner: regular meal

Friday

Breakfast: regular meal

Lunch: regular meal

Dinner: regular meal

The 20:4/Warrior OMAD/23:1 Meal Plan

Although, technically, you could choose any four-hour window in which to eat, *The Warrior Diet*, created by Ori Hofmekler, specifies that the eating window should be in the evening, based on his rationale that our primitive ancestors spent their days hunting, then feasting in the evening. I recommend not eating too late and to try and eat while it is still light out, if possible, to sync your eating with your circadian rhythms.

Although the 20:4/Warrior protocol is based on one main evening meal a day, you have a four-hour window in which to consume it. To do OMAD/23:1, narrow that window to one hour: for example, from 7:00 to 8:00 p.m.

Sample Meal Plan

4:00 pm Starter: Kale Salad with Roasted Sweet Potatoes, Pepitas, and Raspberry Vinaigrette (page 122)

7:00 pm Main: Salmon with Mustard, Maple, and Pecans (page 107)

Sunday

Breakfast: skip

Lunch: skip

Dinner: eat between 4:00 and 8:00 p.m.

Saturday

Breakfast: regular meal

Lunch: regular meal

Dinner: regular meal

Monday

Breakfast: skip

Lunch: skip

Dinner: eat between 4:00 and 8:00 p.m.

Tuesday

Breakfast: skip

Lunch: skip

Dinner: eat between 4:00 and 8:00 p.m.

Wednesday

Breakfast: skip

Lunch: skip

Dinner: eat between 4:00 and
8:00 p.m.

Thursday

Breakfast: skip

Lunch: skip

Dinner: eat between 4:00 and
8:00 p.m.

Friday

Breakfast: skip

Lunch: skip

Dinner: eat between 4:00 and
8:00 p.m.

Saturday

Breakfast: skip

Lunch: skip

Dinner: eat between 4:00 and
8:00 p.m.

The 24-Hour Fast Meal Plan

For this method, you fast once or twice a week for 24 hours. For the remainder of
the week, make sensible, healthy choices. First, choose your 24-hour window. You
could begin by eating dinner at 6:00 p.m. on day one, skipping breakfast and lunch
the next day, and ending your fast with dinner at 6:00 p.m. on day two. Think of
this as skipping two meals in a row—you choose the two meals and you never go
an entire day without eating.

Eating Day Sample Meal Plan

Breakfast: Easy Tofu Scramble
(page 120)

Lunch: Low-Carb Buffalo Chicken
Casserole (page 112)

Dinner: Seared White Fish with
Pan-Fried Vegetables (page 128)

Fasting Day Sample Meal Plan

Dinner: Mediterranean Grilled
Chicken with Lemon Aioli and
Homemade Caesar Salad (page 158)

Sunday

Breakfast: regular meal

Lunch: regular meal

Dinner: regular meal

Monday

Breakfast: regular meal

Lunch: regular meal

Dinner: regular meal

Tuesday

Breakfast: skip

Lunch: skip

Dinner: regular meal

Wednesday

Breakfast: regular meal

Lunch: regular meal

Dinner: regular meal

Thursday

    Breakfast: skip

    Lunch: skip

    Dinner: regular meal

Friday

    Breakfast: regular meal

    Lunch: regular meal

    Dinner: regular meal

Saturday

    Breakfast: regular meal

    Lunch: regular meal

    Dinner: regular meal

The Alternate-Day Meal Plan (Weekly Protocol)

This fasting protocol is straightforward: You fast every other day, either as a clean fast (water, tea, coffee) or a modified fast (about 500–750 calories). The 500–750 calories in your modified fast can be consumed in one to three meals. The sample, I'm providing is two meals. Every other week, switch your fasting days so you don't have two consecutive fasting days. If you prefer to fast on the same days every week, you can choose a 4:3 cycle and keep your fasting days consistent. For example, you can fast every week on Mondays, Wednesdays, and Fridays. Choose the days that work best for you.

Modified Fast with 2 Meals Sample Meal Plan

    Breakfast: Coffee, tea and/or water

    Lunch: Roasted Garlic Cream Soup, 196 calories (page 90)

    Dinner: Spicy Tuna Quinoa Bowl, 307 calories (page 126)

    Total: 513 calories

Eating Day Sample Meal Plan

    Breakfast: Overnight Rolled Oats with Cinnamon (page 116)

    Lunch: Salmon Sandwich with Black Olives and Red Onion (page 146) with a side salad or veggie sticks

    Dinner: Spicy Keto Chicken Tenders with Parmesan Mayo (page 152) served with a side salad

Sunday

Breakfast: water only, or a low-calorie meal

Lunch: water only, or a low-calorie meal

Dinner: water only, or a low-calorie meal

Monday

Breakfast: regular meal

Lunch: regular meal

Dinner: regular meal

Tuesday

Breakfast: water only, or a low-calorie meal

Lunch: water only, or a low-calorie meal

Dinner: water only, or a low-calorie meal

Wednesday

Breakfast: regular meal

Lunch: regular meal

Dinner: regular meal

Thursday

Breakfast: water only, or a low-calorie meal

Lunch: water only, or a low-calorie meal

Dinner: water only, or a low-calorie meal

Friday

Breakfast: regular meal

Lunch: regular meal

Dinner: regular meal

Saturday

Breakfast: water only, or a low-calorie meal

Lunch: water only, or a low-calorie meal

Dinner: water only, or a low-calorie meal

If you choose the water-only option, be sure to read about clean and dirty fasting (see page 62).

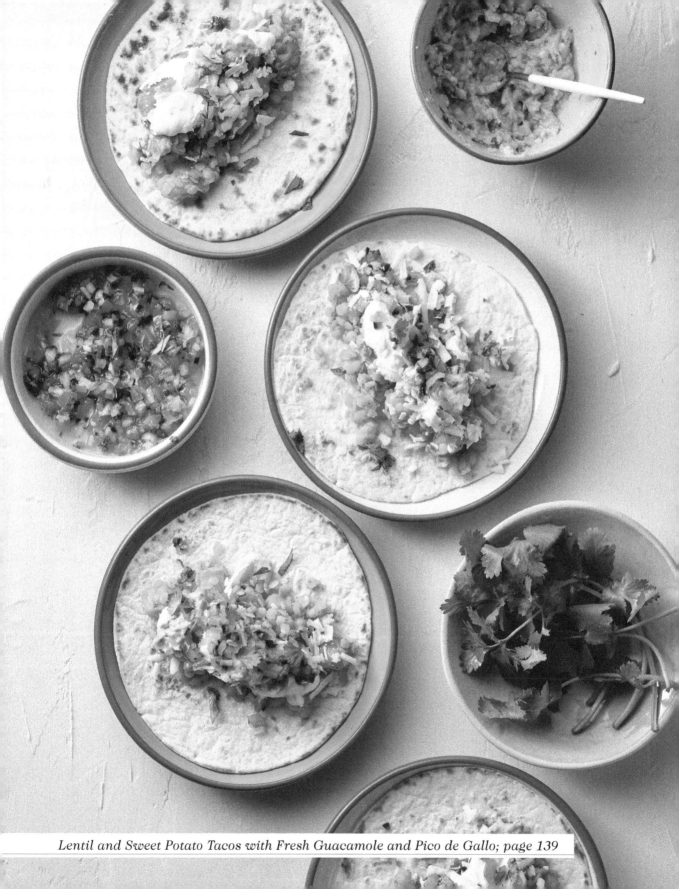

Lentil and Sweet Potato Tacos with Fresh Guacamole and Pico de Gallo; page 139

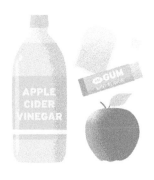

CHAPTER SIX

Fasting Guidance and Challenges

This chapter provides helpful advice for intermittent fasting. Come back to this chapter anytime for a quick reference.

Eating and Drinking Advice for Intermittent Fasting

The advice in this chapter is general. You may have different needs depending on your reason for fasting, so hopefully this chapter addresses them for you.

The Importance of Hydration

According to the National Academies of Sciences, Engineering, and Medicine, drinking water with meals and between meals to satisfy your thirst is enough to meet your needs. When you aren't eating meals, however, you need to replace the water contained *in* the meal as well as the water you would drink *with* the meal. Total fluid needs, including water from all sources, is 3 to 4 quarts per day for adults.

You may want to set reminders for yourself to drink water throughout the day, especially on fasting days. Hydration is crucial for blood pressure control, for healthy kidneys, and to prevent constipation, headaches, and weakness.

What Else You Can Drink While You're Fasting

I want to introduce you to some intermittent fasting lingo: clean fasting and dirty fasting. Clean fasting is stricter, limiting yourself to zero-calorie liquids with zero glucose or insulin response. Dirty fasting allows more options, including items with limited calories such as flavors, artificial and non-nutritive sweeteners, or fat-based calories. The goal is to have a limited rise in glucose. However, it's argued that some foods you eat during a dirty fast, although zero- or low-calorie, may still have an insulin response.

Some fluids you can consume on a clean fast include:

▸ Coffee (no cream, milk, sugar, or sweetener)

▸ Green or black tea (no cream, milk, sugar, or sweetener)

▸ Herbal tea*

▸ Salted water**

▸ Water and sparkling water (no flavor)

*Some herbal teas may elicit a cephalic response (salivating), which could trigger an insulin release in anticipation of food.
**Drinking salted water may help with muscle cramps.

On a dirty fast, you can have:

- Beverages with artificial sweeteners
- Beverages with non-nutritive natural sweeteners (such as monk fruit or stevia)
- Bone Broth (page 92) or other clear broth
- Bulletproof Coffee (page 97) or tea (see tip, page 97)
- Coffee or tea with cream
- Herbal tea
- Pickle juice**
- Sparkling waters with essence (flavoring without sweetener)
- Sugar-free gum
- Water with apple cider vinegar
- Water with lemon, lime, or other fruit infusion

**Drinking salted water may help with muscle cramps.

What is bulletproof coffee (or bulletproof tea)? This is coffee with medium-chain triglyceride oil (MCT oil), butter, coconut oil, or ghee (clarified butter), or some combination of those fats. The fats are whipped into the coffee, resulting in a frothy drink. The idea is that by whipping the fat into the coffee, it's more satiating and can help satisfy hunger. And because there's no sugar and only added fat, it won't take you out of ketosis. (Even if you aren't doing a keto diet, your body will go into ketosis after about 12 hours of fasting.)

There are strict rules on the internet about what's allowed and what isn't allowed in dirty versus clean fasting (for example, unsweetened flavored water isn't allowed on a clean fast, as the flavor is suspected of provoking a cephalic response). Unfortunately, the research studies on fasting can't help shed any light on this subject; you will have to use your best judgment. But understanding this lingo and the rationale behind it can help you be part of the intermittent fasting community that exists.

Do you remember the story of Pavlov and his dogs? Your body can respond to non-nutritive sweeteners in the same way, so when you perceive a flavor and/or sweetness, your body responds with a digestive signal telling your body to expect food. This may cause a release of insulin from the pancreas in anticipation, which would break your fast. This cephalic response occurs even when there are zero calories, like with flavored waters and diet drinks. It may also cause you to feel hungry.

Some people have more difficulty with cravings and hunger when they include diet and low-calorie beverages during fasting. If you have this issue, try clean fasting with just water, coffee, and green or black tea to see whether this helps reduce uncomfortable cravings and hunger and, possibly, even helps with a weight-loss plateau.

People also question whether sweeteners can raise glucose or insulin levels or have other metabolic effects. It's been suggested that non-nutritive sweeteners can elicit a metabolic response by a change in the gut microbiota that triggers glucose intolerance and taste receptors that trigger insulin release. One benefit of fasting is that it can lower insulin levels, so you wouldn't want to consume a sweetener that raises them during your fast.

But can you lose weight with sweeteners? Results are mixed. In a 12-week study, participants drank a beverage sweetened with either sucrose (table sugar), aspartame, saccharin, sucralose, or rebaudioside A. Weight gain occurred with sucrose and saccharin. No weight gain occurred with the other sweeteners, and weight loss only occurred with the sucralose-sweetened beverage.

A 2016 review concluded that if you take a low-energy sweetener in place of sugar, it can lead to reduced calorie intake and body weight. Other research supports weight loss benefits by eliminating sweeteners; in studies that asked diet soda users to switch to water, the participants lost more weight and had lower insulin and insulin resistance levels.

Although the proponents of dirty and clean fasting have strong feelings about their approaches, currently, we don't have research that supports one type of fast over the other.

You don't need to consume a low-calorie sweetener; they're optional and you can be just as successful on IF, if not more so, if you avoid them. Experiment and observe your results. Similarly, experiment with dirty and clean fasting. If you struggle with cravings, hunger, or a weight-loss plateau, try clean fasting. If you need something to help you get through your fast, try coffee with cream, Bone Broth (page 92), or Bulletproof Coffee (page 97).

About Snacking

Eating more frequently has been thought to increase metabolism, reduce hunger, improve glucose and insulin control, and reduce body weight. But research is inconclusive on this. Without research to guide a recommendation, it really comes down to self-observation. For example, if you choose an eight-hour eating window—such as 12:00 to 8:00 p.m.—you may choose to eat lunch and dinner only or to have lunch, an afternoon snack, dinner, and an after-dinner snack. You may find that eating an afternoon snack allows you to eat a smaller dinner and not snack again in the evening. If you're hungry after your feeding window has closed, drink water, coffee, or tea. If it's late, you may prefer decaf.

Your Social Life When Fasting

You *can* have a social life and family life while fasting. I'll offer some helpful advice.

Dining Out

When eating out:

- If you are on a modified fasting day, check the menu for calorie information, or check the restaurant's website before you go to help guide your choices.
- After eating out, pay attention to your feeling of hunger before your next scheduled meal; you may choose to skip the next meal or reduce it, especially if the restaurant meal was bigger or richer than usual.
- If you overdo it, get back on track for your next meal.
- It's okay to be flexible to avoid awkward situations. In fact, being flexible will help you maintain IF in the long term.

Meals with Your Family

Research supports that eating meals as a family has many benefits, including providing structure for the day, better nutrition, lower frequency of disordered eating, lower drug use and other high-risk behaviors in teens, and better relationships with family members. It's often recommended that families have at least one meal together per day—for many of us, this meal is dinner.

So, how do you have a family meal while fasting? Ideally, you can plan your fast so you're able to eat with the family. Most IF regimens allow at least one meal a day. If you can't eat a full meal, see whether you can have something different than the rest of the family, like a clear soup. Maybe breakfast together works better than dinner. Be creative and do your best to maintain family meal traditions.

Holidays

Not surprisingly, holidays present their own set of challenges. Your best bet? Plan for them. You may need to get creative with your eating windows and adjust the times to accommodate a holiday meal and extend the next day's fast. Trying to fast as a guest at someone's home may unintentionally offend your host, so consider extending your fast before the event to allow you to eat or giving your host a heads-up ahead of time so they understand your situation. If it's a dinner party, offer to bring a big dish of something you know you can eat and share it with others.

Telling Others You're Fasting

What information to share and who to share it with is a personal choice. It's helpful to have support. If you expect someone to support you with your fasting, be clear about what you need from them.

You may also choose not to share, especially if you expect there may be some sabotage at play. Some examples of sabotage could include statements from others, such as:

- "But it's my birthday!"
- "I got this for you because I know it's your favorite. Just eat it!"
- "You can't be good all the time!"
- "You need to have a cheat day once in a while."

Although friends and family love us, sometimes others can see our progress as leaving them behind. It's not that they don't want you to succeed—they may be self-conscious of their own inaction. Try not to take sabotage personally; it's more about them and how they feel about themselves than it is about you.

You may find that people respond better when you frame your change as a health goal rather than purely weight loss. For example, "I need to get my blood sugar down," rather than, "I want to lose weight." Communicating your goals in this way may help them be better received and trigger fewer feelings of shame in others that can result in sabotage.

What to Say to Your Doctor

You'll want to be open with your doctor, especially if you'll require extra monitoring during intermittent fasting. If your doctor has concerns, listen carefully and do your best to mitigate those concerns with the regimen you choose.

To minimize risks associated with intermittent fasting, you can advise your doctor that you're slowly easing into IF, staying hydrated, continuing your medication, and choosing the best method for your concerns. You can also show them the References section in this book (page 174). Your doctor may suggest you work with a registered dietitian who can monitor your diet and advise you while you fast.

IS FASTING DIFFERENT FOR MEN AND WOMEN?

Throughout this section, specific gender vocabulary will be used. This is not intended to exclude, offend, or alienate, but simply to take a straightforward approach when explaining how fasting uniquely targets the cisgender woman and her unique physiology.

There is limited research on this topic. Gender influences metabolic rates, so it helps to know how female physiology can work for or against health goals. On social media, I've seen both the recommendation that women should not do longer fasts (more than 14 hours), as it is "too stressful to the adrenals and thyroid," and that they should do longer fasts (20 hours plus), as the "body thrives in a fasted state," but neither was backed up by research. Popular media say women have lower metabolic rates than men and an article in the *Journal of Applied Physiology* demonstrates that this basic concept is backed up scientifically due to several main factors, two of which are body mass and hormones.

Body mass refers to your overall weight and size, which can promote or decrease metabolism. Males are typically larger than females, giving men a biologically higher metabolic rate.

When it comes to hormones, testosterone promotes higher muscle tissue, whereas estrogen promotes fat storage. Estrogen specifically promotes the storage of subcutaneous fat, which sits away from organs on breasts, glutes, and thighs and sustains the body's reproductive potential. Men's bodies tend to have a higher distribution of visceral fat. The hormones that work to regulate fat, muscle, and metabolic rate for women fluctuate, which can lead to changes in fat storage and shifting metabolic levels. These biological differences give men a slight advantage for having a naturally higher metabolism, but that doesn't mean women can't have similar metabolic levels. Fasting can be a tool for women looking to create a more efficient metabolism without throwing their hormones out of whack.

In addition to this, due to the differences in sex hormones and gender distributions of adipose tissue, women tend to have a higher risk of insulin resistance and lower fat-burning capabilities than men.

Women may also experience changes to their menstrual cycle while fasting. I've seen anecdotal reports of women without a menstrual cycle getting one back with IF. If this is you, be aware that this could mean you may be able to become pregnant when you previously thought you could not. Discuss with your doctor whether IF is a good plan while trying to become pregnant. Presently, intermittent fasting is not recommended if you are currently pregnant, breastfeeding, or underweight.

On a side note: Women should target an intake of 18 grams of iron a day because they lose it through menstruation. When you're not fasting, focus on consuming iron-rich foods. If you take a multivitamin-mineral, make sure it is for younger women, so it has the higher iron levels. If you are concerned, have your blood levels checked with your family physician.

Lastly, as women age, estrogen production declines and bone loss accelerates, putting women at greater risk of brittle bones and osteoporosis. To promote health, focus on whole foods, like dairy and leafy greens, to get an adequate calcium intake. To measure your bone density, you can request a bone scan, especially if your bone structure is petite or if there is a family history of osteoporosis.

Simply put, women are different from men; women are different from each other; your pre-pregnancy self is different from your post-pregnancy self; and your premenopausal self is different from your postmenopausal self. Use trial and error to find the best intermittent fasting schedule for you. Don't feel that more is better and that you're "not doing it right" if a shorter fast is where you settle in. Typically, women are slower to lose weight than men, so try not to compare your results with others. A good rule of thumb for anyone is to start slowly and listen to your body. If you feel truly lousy (not just hungry), discontinue fasting and consider seeing a medical professional for guidance.

Fasting If You Have Diabetes

As discussed previously, research has shown overweight and obese adults with type 2 diabetes who followed 5:2 (with mostly nonconsecutive days and a minimum of 50 grams of protein per day) showed improvement in blood sugar control similar to those on continuous calorie restriction.

In a study comparing whether consecutive or nonconsecutive days of 5:2 fasting resulted in fewer low blood sugars, researchers found no difference. In this study, sulfonylureas and insulins were adjusted as follows:

- Apidra, Humalog, Humulin R, and NovoRapid were reduced by 70 percent on fasting days.
- Lantus was reduced by 50 percent the morning of a fasting day and/or by 50 percent the evening before a fasting day.
- Metformin and other nonhypoglycemia-causing medications were not changed.
- Mixed insulins were reduced by 25 percent the night before a fast and 50 percent the day of a fast.
- NPH insulins were reduced by 50 percent on fasting days.

Despite these changes, 59 percent of participants experienced one low blood sugar for every 37 days of fasting (and one low blood sugar for every 75 days of nonfasting). There was one low blood sugar for every 43 days of consecutive fasts and one for every 80 days for nonconsecutive fasting. None of the hypoglycemia events were severe. Several participants required further adjustments to their diabetes medication. There were double the low blood sugar episodes during fasting compared with nonfasting, but fewer than expected. The participants had weekly monitoring by a physician and were successful in losing weight.

Fasting If You Are Prediabetic

If you're prediabetic, research suggests your insulin sensitivity will improve and your insulin levels will go down, even if you don't lose weight. A reduction in blood pressure and evening appetite can also be expected. As a common benefit of intermittent fasting, weight loss would also benefit prediabetes and help reduce the risk of it progressing to full diabetes.

Fasting and the Keto Diet

Fasting and keto can both put the body into ketosis. Although a ketogenic diet keeps the body in ketosis, intermittent fasting cycles in and out of ketosis. You can combine IF with keto; starting with one then adding the other is a sensible approach. You don't need to do keto when you're intermittent fasting, but if you choose to, there are great keto recipes in this book (see chapter 12). If you are already on a keto diet, IF may help boost your ketone levels.

On the ketogenic diet, macronutrients are key. Keeping dietary carbs, fat, and protein in the right proportions keeps insulin low and cues up ketosis.

Fat is the main macronutrient on keto. It helps build cell membranes, absorb fat-soluble vitamins, and make ketones. Of all the macronutrients, fat raises insulin the least, helping the body stay in ketosis.

You need the building blocks of protein to form nearly every tissue in your body, including muscle. With ketogenic diets though, you aim to get enough protein to meet your needs, but not more. It's a moderate protein diet, not a high protein diet.

Low-carb means low blood sugar, low blood sugar means low insulin, and low insulin means fat-burning.

Lastly: you might want to try IF first instead of trying keto and IF at the same time. Try a month or two of IF as an initial step—it might help make the transition into combined IF and keto smoother.

Fasting When You Have a Low Tolerance for High Fat

Intermittent fasting doesn't need to be paired with a low-carb/high-fat diet. The beauty of IF is you can eat normally. I also included recipes that are low-fat in chapter 10.

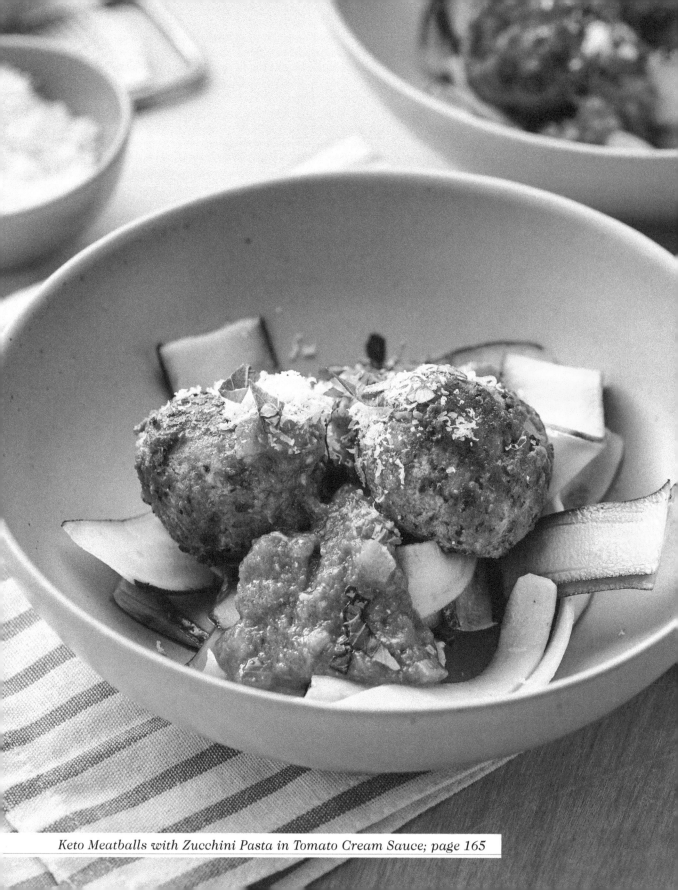

Keto Meatballs with Zucchini Pasta in Tomato Cream Sauce; page 165

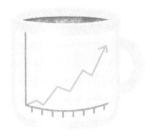

CHAPTER SEVEN

Taking Fasting to the Next Level

This section tackles everything else you'll want to know, including how to maintain and advance your fasting lifestyle.

Maintaining an Intermittent-Fasting Lifestyle

Ideally, you should consider intermittent fasting as a lifestyle, not a diet. Although there's limited data on long-term use of intermittent fasting, research continues. Intermittent fasting appears to provide a sustainable version of caloric restriction, which is linked to longevity.

What Long-Term Fasting Looks Like

Although I read more than 90 scientific publications in my research for this book, the longest trial I found was 18 months with humans and another with a two-year follow-up. I'm not able to say with certainty what you can expect when you continue your intermittent-fasting lifestyle for years, but like much of IF, there's plenty of room for self-exploration.

As a registered dietitian, I have a concern about micronutrient deficiencies. It's uncertain, if you restrict yourself to one meal a day for years, whether you be able to get all the vitamins, minerals, and fiber you need for optimal health. However, you can help increase the likelihood that you will by choosing whole, unprocessed foods. For long-term maintenance, having two meals or a meal and a snack will give you a better opportunity to receive the nutrition you need from food without relying on supplements, especially if you have a medical condition that limits your body's ability to digest or absorb nutrients.

Having yearly blood work and regular bone density scans are strategies you can discuss with your physician to monitor your health. Although getting your nutrition from food is preferred, you may also want to take a multivitamin-mineral supplement.

If you want to continue IF for the long term, be flexible to prevent feelings of deprivation or missing out while maintaining your goals. For example, you may find that rather than 18:6 every day, you do 18:6 Sunday to Thursday and 16:8 on the weekends. You might have no fasting on the weekend, 24-hour fasts on Mondays, and 72-hour fasts once a month. The combinations are endless, and there's no one right way to fast—other than safely.

Dropping Out . . . and Back In

If you feel as though you just can't stick with intermittent fasting and you need a break, make the decision to stop when you aren't hungry or at your worst. Before dropping out, try addressing these issues:

If you're getting too hungry: Reduce the length of your fast. Even a 12:12 window is a form of intermittent fasting.

If you're craving: Pay attention to potential triggers. Are you seeing tempting foods on the counter? Are you being triggered when you watch TV? Are you watching other people eat? Is sugar-free gum, diet soda, or your brand of toothpaste making you crave? Try a multivitamin-mineral to rule out micronutrient deficiencies as a possible cause. Are cravings triggered by worry, fear, or boredom? If so, implement a solution that targets these triggers. Are you craving out of habit? If so, change your routine. If you're craving sweets, try reducing your carbs in your eating window. If you're dirty fasting, try clean fasting. If you're clean fasting, see whether dirty fasting with Bone Broth (page 92) or Bulletproof Coffee (page 97) helps, but stay away from sweeteners, even zero-calorie ones.

If you're finding social situations difficult: Try fasting on some days and not others. Or have different feeding/fasting windows on different days. Although it might take a little longer to reach your goal, you're still moving in the right direction.

If you aren't getting support: Find support from others who are fasting. Intermittent-fasting groups can provide support and encouragement during these times (see page 171). If you need to, find a registered dietitian who has experience with fasting.

If you have multiple health issues: Work with a health professional to prioritize which issue to focus on first and determine the best strategy.

If you're stuck in a weight-loss plateau: Try a different eating window. Shortening or lengthening an eating window can help. Try some extended fasts. Alternately, try shifting the window earlier in the day to focus on eating during peak daylight hours. Try adding low-intensity exercise just before you open your window to maximize fat burn.

If you feel that fasting is just not working, it's okay to take a break. It'll be here for you when you're ready to try again. When you're ready to return, you should start from the beginning and not jump back to where you were when you stopped to minimize side-effects.

Why You Might Decide to Advance to Extended Fasting

Once you have some fasting experience, you might want to try different protocols. You might be especially drawn to this if you find yourself on a plateau.

I suggest you graduate to this in steps. For example, if you're doing a 16:8, move to 18:6 then 20:4. You can also try 24-hour fasts, OMAD, alternate-daily fasting, or 36-hour fasting. Once you have experience with these, you can try an extended fast beyond 48 hours. Extending your fasting is an option, but it's not a necessary progression. Extended fasts should be done under medical supervision.

How to Take on an Extended Fast

Before you prepare for an extended fast, be clear on why you're doing it, what you hope to achieve, how to set yourself up for success, and what signal would indicate you're ready to end the fast.

Decide if it will be water only or if you'll follow a dirty fast or modified fast. *Dry fasting (without water) is not recommended.*

Pick a few uneventful regular days for your first extended fast. I don't recommend extended fasting during days when parties, work events, or new or taxing activities are scheduled.

You might find it easier to fast at the end of a grocery cycle, but make sure you have plenty of your favorite fasting beverages on hand. You may find your transition easier if you reduce your carbohydrate intake in the day(s) before you begin. If you're testing ketones or blood sugar, have your keto sticks or glucometer test strips available.

Otherwise, the preparation is mostly mental. You may want to plan activities or projects to help divert your attention during hunger pangs.

The hunger hormone ghrelin peaks at 18 hours, meaning you'll be hungriest then. This will help you calculate when to begin your fast. For example, if you begin your fast after breakfast, 18 hours later you'll be asleep during the hunger peak. However, there's still a lot of trial and error involved.

If you experience low blood sugar, keep a fast-acting sugar on hand when you're away from home. If you take medication, talk to your doctor or pharmacist about what changes might be needed for your usual dosages and what side effects to expect.

Here are some potential issues with extended fasts:

Muscle cramps and headaches. These could signal low sodium and other electrolytes. Bone Broth (page 92), salted water, or pickle juice can provide sodium. If these liquids taste good to you, you're likely low in sodium.

Elevated uric acids levels. Uric acid is responsible for the painful joint condition known as gout. If you have gout, it doesn't mean you can't do extended fasts, but you'll need to consider the risks and benefits and discuss monitoring your uric acid levels with your doctor.

Gallstone formation. One study showed that people who are obese who lose weight rapidly are at increased risk of gallstone formation. However, it was also noted that when weight loss was from fasting, the cholesterol saturation went down. To assess your risk, discuss testing your cholesterol saturation or having an ultrasound of your gallbladder with your physician. Aspirin and ursodeoxycholic acid were shown to reduce the risk of gallstone development as well.

Refeeding syndrome. This condition can occur with longer fasts and usually targets lower-weight and underweight individuals. It's a shift in fluid and electrolytes that can cause edema and low blood levels of phosphorus and other electrolytes two to five days after carbohydrates are reintroduced. It can be dangerous and is the reason medical supervision is recommended for extended fasts. The recommendation to prevent refeeding syndrome is to "start low, advance slow" when you break your fast. In refeeding patients with anorexia, the recommendation to prevent refeeding syndrome is to begin with 600 to 1,000 calories per day and to increase 300 to 400 calories every three to four days. Use that as a guide to help you successfully reintroduce food after an extended fast.

For longer fasts and food reintroduction, I recommend monitoring your heart rate, edema, weight regain, and bowel routine. I also suggest discussing the risks and benefits and the plan with your physician before you undertake an extended fast. There's little research to guide us on this, so extended fasts must be individualized.

10 Ways to Biohack

Biohacking is described as "do-it-yourself biology" and, generally, consists of making small incremental changes to improve your health and well-being. Intermittent fasting is considered a biohack, as early evidence points to longevity benefits. Here are some other biohacks you can add to your routine:

1. Get a good night's sleep. Sleep is profoundly restorative for many systems in our body, including the immune system. Cold showers can help you sleep better, too.

2. Spend time in nature. Research from Japan has shown an increase in certain disease-fighting white blood cells after people spend time in nature. *Shinrin-yoku*, or forest bathing, is the name of the practice (see Resources, page 171).

3. Spice it up. As a dietitian specializing in cancer risk reduction, I often read about the benefits of a plant-based diet. Herbs and spices are an important, often-overlooked part of that diet. I challenge you to use at least one herb or spice with every meal!

4. Move regularly. Even if you get a good workout in the morning, sitting all day is not ideal. Try to get up once an hour and move.

5. Spend quality time with others. Although this recommendation has its challenges (at the time of writing, we're dealing with Covid-19 and social distancing), find ways to make safe connections.

6. Quiet your brain. Even 10 minutes a day of quiet reflection can help restore your mind-body connection.

7. Laugh! Laughing increases immune cells and is linked to a decrease in all-cause mortality and cardiovascular disease.

8. Nourish your body. Even though IF is all about when you eat, try to eat real, whole foods, not processed foods.

9. Focus on health, not just weight. Weight does not always go down as expected with IF. Many people report other benefits such as reduced size, clearer skin, improved energy, and less pain. Look for and acknowledge those rewards for your efforts, too. In social media, these are called nonscale victories, or NSVs.

10. Reclaim your time. By doing intermittent fasting, you'll gain back time you would normally use to prepare and eat meals. Don't let that time get eaten up by the general business of your day. Use it for something that brings you joy.

PART THREE

What to Eat (When You Do Eat)

Eating is as important to intermittent fasting as the fasting is! Most of the recipes in this section will be for your feeding window, but I also include several that can be consumed as part of a dirty fast or during a modified fasting day. I divide the recipes into five sections, based on different needs. You should be able to find exactly what you need by chapter title.

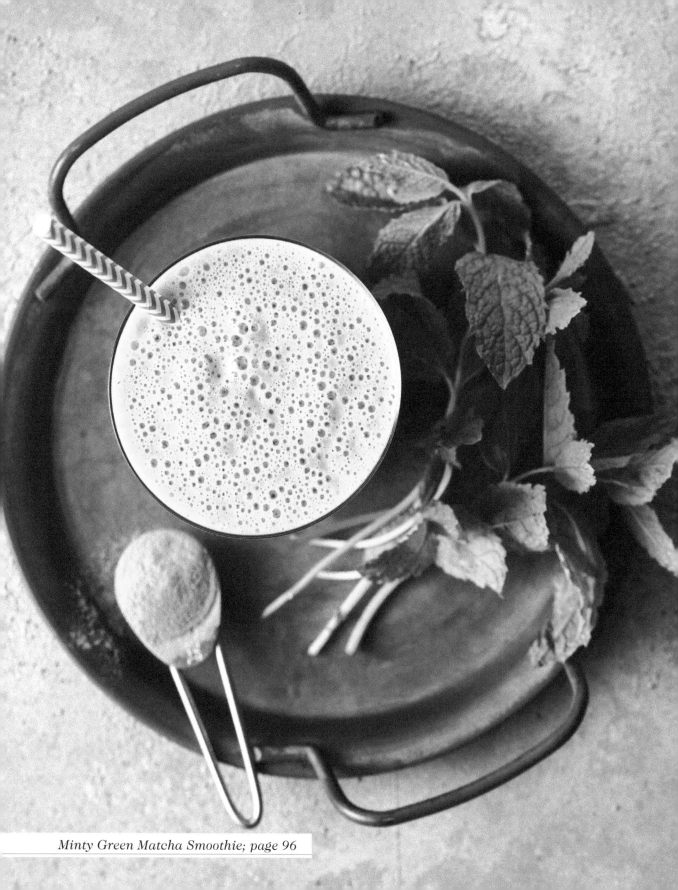

Minty Green Matcha Smoothie; page 96

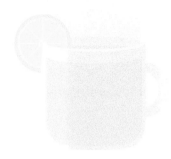

CHAPTER EIGHT

Broths and Drinks

If there's one takeaway as you begin fasting, it's this: Stay hydrated! These recipes can be used as part of your dirty fast, modified fast, or on feeding days. If the soup is strained, the broth can be used for dirty fasting; if it is served without straining, then most can be used for modified fasting, and if it is served with added items, like the avocado cream, it's only for your feeding window.

Lemony Chicken Broth

Prep time: 10 minutes / **Cook time:** 35 minutes
Serves: 4
Clean Eating, Low-Calorie, Low-Carb, Low-Fat, One Pot

This recipe is versatile—strain it and enjoy the broth as part of your dirty fast, or leave the vegetables and cube the chicken for a low-carb meal (see tip). It's satisfying and flavorful and comes together quickly.

1 tablespoon extra-virgin
  olive oil
1 onion, diced
2 carrots, diced
1 celery stalk, halved
  lengthwise and diced
2 garlic cloves, minced
3 skin-on chicken legs
4 cups chicken broth
  or water, plus more if
  needed, divided
½ teaspoon dried thyme
Juice of 1 lemon, plus
  more as needed
½ teaspoon salt
Freshly ground
  black pepper

1. In a large pot over medium heat, heat the oil. Add the onion and cook for 3 to 4 minutes, stirring, until softened.

2. Add the carrots, celery, and garlic. Cook for 6 to 8 minutes, stirring occasionally, until the vegetables are soft and caramelized.

3. Add the chicken legs. Cook the chicken for 3 to 5 minutes, until browned and they stick to the pot. Turn the chicken a quarter turn and pour in ¼ cup of chicken broth to deglaze the pot, stirring to scrape up any browned bits from the bottom. Continue to brown the chicken and deglaze the pot with ¼ cup of broth at each turn, until the chicken is browned all over.

4. Add the remaining 3 cups of broth, increase the heat to medium-high and bring to a boil. Cook the chicken for 10 to 15 minutes more, until the chicken is cooked through. Add more broth if the soup is getting too thick.

5. Stir in the thyme and lemon juice. Taste and add more lemon juice if desired, and the salt and pepper to taste.

6. Strain the soup through a colander set over a heat-proof bowl and enjoy the broth.

Variation tip: If you want a low-carb soup, after straining the soup, transfer the chicken to a cutting board. Remove the skin and discard. Remove the chicken meat, cut it into cubes, and return it to the soup.

Per Serving: Calories: 166; Total Fat: 10g; Total Carbs: 5g; Fiber: 1g; Sugar: 3g; Protein 13g; Sodium: 1268mg

Herbed Turkey Broth

Prep time: 15 minutes / **Cook time:** 40 minutes
Serves: 4
Clean Eating, Low-Calorie, Low-Carb, Low-Fat, One Pot

Sage, rosemary, and thyme are the herbs I use to make stuffing at Thanksgiving, so by using these as part of the poultry seasoning, it reminds me of eating a satisfying roast turkey meal with all the fixins! Enjoy the broth as a dirty fast, or have the soup as a low-carb dish (see tip).

1 tablespoon extra-virgin olive oil

1 onion, diced

1 celery stalk, diced

2 carrots, diced

1 skin-on turkey leg (about 1 pound)

8 cups water, divided

1 teaspoon salt, plus more as needed

1 teaspoon dried rosemary leaves, crushed

½ teaspoon dried thyme

½ teaspoon dried sage

Nutmeg

Freshly ground black pepper

Chopped fresh parsley, for garnish (optional)

1. In a medium pot over medium-low heat, heat the oil. Add the onion, celery, and carrots. Increase the heat to medium and cook for about 5 minutes, stirring occasionally, or until the vegetables are softened.

2. Add the turkey leg. Cook for 3 to 5 minutes, until the vegetables and turkey stick to the pot. Pour in ¼ cup of water to deglaze the pot, stirring to scrape up any browned bits from the bottom. Turn the turkey leg a quarter turn and repeat the browning and deglazing with ¼ cup of water three more times. The turkey leg should appear browned all over.

3. Transfer the turkey leg to a cutting board and remove and discard the skin. Return the turkey leg to the pot.

4. Add the remaining 7 cups of water, increase the heat to medium-high, and bring to a boil. Reduce the heat to medium.

5. Stir in the salt, rosemary, thyme, sage, and a pinch of nutmeg. Cook for 10 minutes more, or until the turkey reaches an internal temperature of 165°F.

6. Strain the broth through a colander set over a heatproof bowl and enjoy the broth. Taste and season with more salt and pepper as needed. Top with the parsley (if using).

Variation tip: For a low-carb soup, after straining the broth, transfer the turkey leg to a cutting board. Remove the meat, cut it into cubes, and return it to the soup.

Per Serving: Calories: 159; Total Fat: 9g; Total Carbs: 3g; Fiber: 1g; Sugar: 1g; Protein 17g; Sodium: 648mg

Cilantro Lime Broth with Avocado Cream

Prep time: 20 minutes / **Cook time:** 15 minutes
Serves: 2
Low-Calorie, Low-Carb, Low-Fat

This is the fasting version of a traditional Peruvian soup recipe, modified to keep it low-carb and low-insulinemic but still flavorful. The optional avocado cream increases the fat content and makes this soup more satiating.

For the broth

1 garlic clove, peeled

1 tablespoon extra-virgin olive oil

1 small onion, chopped

1 jalapeño pepper, finely diced

4 cups low-sodium chicken broth

1 cup tightly packed fresh cilantro leaves

3 tablespoons freshly squeezed lime juice (from about 3 limes)

¾ teaspoon salt

For the avocado cream (optional)

1 large ripe avocado, halved and pitted

¼ cup sour cream

1½ teaspoons freshly squeezed lime juice

1 teaspoon finely minced fresh cilantro leaves

½ teaspoon salt

To make the broth

1. Mince the garlic and let it sit for 10 minutes.

2. In a medium pot over medium heat, heat the oil. Add the onion and cook for 4 to 5 minutes, stirring occasionally. Reduce the heat to medium-low and add the garlic and jalapeño. Cook for about 5 minutes, stirring, until softened, being careful not to burn the garlic.

3. Add the chicken broth to deglaze the pot, stirring to scrape up any browned bits from the bottom. Increase the heat to medium-high. Cook for 5 to 10 minutes.

4. In a food processor, process the cilantro leaves until pureed. Add the chicken broth mixture, lime juice, and salt. Pulse to combine. Transfer to a large bowl and clean the food processor.

To make the avocado cream (if using)

5. Scoop the avocado flesh into a food processor and add the sour cream, lime juice, cilantro, and salt. Process until smooth, stopping to scrape down the sides as needed.

6. Spoon the soup into shallow bowls and top with the avocado cream (if using).

Addition tip: If you want this broth to be more substantial, add 1 cup of pulled or cubed cooked chicken to the broth.

Per Serving: Calories: 343; Total Fat: 28g; Total Carbs: 20g; Fiber: 8g; Sugar: 6g; Protein 6g; Sodium: 1726mg

Roasted Garlic Cream Soup

Prep time: 10 minutes / **Cook time:** about 1 hour
Serves: 4
Low-Calorie, Low-Carb

When you cut a garlic clove, you expose two compounds previously separated within their own membranes. These chemicals come together to form allicin. If you let cut garlic sit on the cutting board for 10 minutes before cooking, you maximize the conversion of allicin to other important cancer-fighting compounds.

3 garlic heads (about
  45 cloves)
1 tablespoon extra-virgin
  olive oil
4 cups chicken broth
¼ teaspoon red
  pepper flakes
½ cup heavy
  (whipping) cream
1 teaspoon salt
  (if using low-sodium
  broth; optional)

1. Preheat the oven to 400°F.

2. Tear off a 12-inch-long piece of aluminum foil. Remove some loose skin from the garlic heads. Cut the garlic heads horizontally across the middle. (If using hardneck garlic, remove the hard wooden center piece and discard.) Place the garlic halves, cut-side up, on the foil. Drizzle the garlic with the oil, then wrap them in the foil. Place the foil pack in the oven.

3. Bake for 40 to 50 minutes. The garlic is done when it's soft and slightly darker in color.

4. Place the chicken broth in a blender.

5. Using a small fork, carefully remove the roasted garlic cloves from their skins and add them to the blender. Blend until smooth. Transfer the roasted garlic puree to a medium pot and add the red pepper flakes. Place the pot over medium-high heat and bring to a low boil. Cook for 10 to 15 minutes.

6. Reduce the heat, stir in the heavy cream, and cook for 2 to 3 minutes, until heated through. Taste and season with salt as needed.

Variation tip: Omit the cream.

Per Serving: Calories: 196; Total Fat: 15g; Total Carbs: 13g; Fiber: 1g; Sugar: 2g; Protein 5g; Sodium: 938mg

Miso Broth

Prep time: 10 minutes
Serves: 2
5 Ingredients or Less, 30 Minutes or Less, Clean Eating, Low-Calorie, Low-Carb, Low-Fat

Miso is made by fermenting soybeans with rice, barley, or wheat to create a paste. The darker the color, the longer the fermentation and the stronger the flavor. White miso has a milder, slightly sweet flavor, whereas red miso has a stronger umami (savory meat) flavor. Awase miso is a mixture of red and white, making it a versatile condiment. For this broth, I use a white/light miso. Experiment to find the one you like best.

2 tablespoons white miso

3 cups hot water, divided

1 (0.16-ounce) package nori seaweed, crumbled

1 scallion, chopped

1. Place 1 tablespoon of miso into each of two bowls. Add 1½ cups of boiling water to each and stir to dissolve.

2. Top each with the crumbled seaweed and chopped scallion.

Craving tip: If you're craving salt, add soy sauce.

Per Serving: Calories: 41; Total Fat: <1g; Total Carbs: 6g; Fiber: 3g; Sugar: 3g; Protein 3g; Sodium: 478mg

Bone Broth

Prep time: 10 minutes / **Cook time:** 9 hours, plus 4 or more hours to chill
Makes: 5 cups
Low-Calorie, Low-Carb Low-Fat

Broth is usually made from meat, whereas bone broth is made from meaty joints and bones. This classic Bone Broth can be used during your dirty fast or on a modified fasting day, or to open up your fasting window. You may find the minerals in this broth helpful in warding off headaches and muscle cramps. For this recipe, I went to my local butcher and bought a bag of beef knuckle bones and 2 raw chicken carcasses. You can save your bones from a beef, chicken, or pork roast and use those, too.

2 chicken carcasses
(1½ to 2 pounds)
2½ to 3 pounds
beef bones
1 gallon water, plus more
as needed
2 tablespoons apple
cider vinegar
2 onions, halved
1 carrot, quartered
1 celery stalk, quartered
6 peppercorns
½ teaspoon salt

1. Preheat the oven to 400°F. Line a baking sheet with parchment paper.

2. Place the chicken carcasses and beef bones on the prepared baking sheet.

3. Bake for 20 minutes. Transfer the bones to a large stockpot. Add the water and vinegar. Let sit for 20 minutes.

4. Place the pot over high heat and bring the water to a boil. Add the onions, carrot, celery, and peppercorns. Reduce the heat to maintain a simmer and cook for 8 hours. Remove any foam or residue that rises to the surface and add water periodically as the level goes down to bring it back up above the bones.

5. Strain the broth through a colander set over a heatproof bowl. Cover and refrigerate the broth overnight.

6. The next morning, skim the fat from the top of the broth and discard.

7. Return the broth to a pot and gently warm on the stovetop. Taste and season with salt as needed.

Variation tip: Enjoy the bone broth on its own or use it to flavor soup recipes.

Make-ahead tip: Portion the bone broth into individual servings and refrigerate for up to 4 or 5 days, or freeze it for up to 1 year.

Per Serving (1 to 1½ cups): Calories: 57; Total Fat: 3g; Total Carbs: 4g; Fiber: 1g; Sugar: 2g; Protein 5g; Sodium: 312mg

Almond Smoothie with Dates and Cinnamon

Prep time: 10 minutes
Serves: 1
30 Minutes or Less, Clean Eating

Are you having a sweet craving but avoiding refined sugars? This almond-date smoothie is just the thing to satisfy that craving. The sweetness comes from the dates, but we slow down the blood sugar rise by combining it with the healthy fats and protein in almond butter and improve the insulin response with a generous addition of cinnamon.

5 small to medium dates
Hot water, for soaking
  the dates
1 cup unsweetened
  soy milk
1 banana
½ cup almond butter
½ teaspoon ground
  cinnamon, divided
1½ teaspoons maple
  syrup (optional)

1. Place the dates in a small bowl and add enough hot water to cover. Let sit for about 3 minutes to soften. Drain. Remove and discard the pits.

2. In a blender, combine the softened dates, soy milk, banana, almond butter, and ¼ teaspoon of cinnamon. Blend until mixed. Taste and add the remaining cinnamon and maple syrup (if using).

Variation tip: Craving chocolate? Make it a Chocolate-Hazelnut Smoothie. Swap the almond butter for hazelnut butter, use only ⅛ teaspoon of ground cinnamon, and add 5 teaspoons of cocoa powder to the remaining ingredients. Follow the recipe as directed.

Refrigerate the smoothie overnight to gel and enjoy it as a pudding.

Almond Smoothie with Dates and Cinnamon, Per Serving: Calories: 1056; Total Fat: 74g; Total Carbs: 82g; Fiber: 22g; Sugar: 44g; Protein 35g; Sodium: 86mg

Chocolate-Hazelnut Smoothie, Per Serving: Calories: 921; Total Fat: 69g; Total Carbs: 56g; Fiber: 24g; Sugar: 24g; Protein 30g; Sodium: 78mg

Green Zinger Shot

Prep time: 10 minutes
Makes: 12 ounces
30 Minutes or Less, Clean Eating, Low-Fat, One Pot

This is my neighbor's recipe—and it's potent! One shot of this and I feel like I've just had a phytonutrient cocktail. A little goes a long way. You'll see what I mean—the ginger and lemon are a big wake-up call.

1 large apple, halved
  and cored
½ cup tightly packed
  chopped kale
½ cup tightly packed fresh
  baby spinach
5 tablespoons freshly
  squeezed lemon juice
2 teaspoons minced
  peeled fresh ginger
1½ teaspoons honey
1 cup water

1. In a high-speed blender, combine the apple, kale, spinach, lemon juice, ginger, honey, and water. Blend until smooth. Let sit for 5 to 15 minutes to allow the flavors to combine.

2. Serve in a shot glass or small tumbler. Refrigerate, covered, for up to 3 days.

Craving tip: You might find this is just the thing to bust a sweet craving or to open your feeding window.

Per Serving (1½ ounces): Calories: 177; Total Fat: 1g;
Total Carbs: 46g; Fiber: 7g; Sugar: 34g; Protein 2g; Sodium: 22mg

Minty Green Matcha Smoothie

Prep time: 5 minutes
Serves: 1
5 Ingredients or Less, 30 Minutes or Less, Clean Eating, Low-Fat, One Pot

Matcha is made by finely grinding green tea leaves into powder. It tastes like green tea but is very versatile in recipes. This smoothie provides a real morning pick-me-up with its green tea flavor, caffeine, and a refreshing hint of mint.

1 banana
1 teaspoon matcha green
   tea powder
1½ cups unsweetened
   soy milk
2 to 5 drops food-grade
   peppermint oil, or
   8 to 12 fresh mint leaves

In a blender, combine the banana, matcha, soy milk, and peppermint oil or mint leaves. Blend until smooth. Taste, adding more mint as needed.

Ingredient tip: Some peppermint oils are very strong. To prevent your smoothie from tasting like mouthwash, start with less, taste, then gently add more, if needed. Record the amount you used so you'll know for next time.

Variation tip: If you're out of bananas, substitute 2 teaspoons of honey for sweetness. If you have a Magic Bullet, it makes it nice and frothy!

Variation tip: Choose whichever milk you prefer. I use soy milk because it's the highest in protein of all the plant milks. I also appreciate the beneficial immune-supportive attributes of the isoflavones. The latest research shows that soy intake is associated with reduced recurrence of breast cancer. Because soy is approved for genetic modification, you may feel more comfortable with an organic soy beverage.

Per Serving: Calories: 230; Total Fat: 6g; Total Carbs: 33g; Fiber: 6g; Sugar: 16g; Protein 14g; Sodium: 114mg

Bulletproof Coffee

Prep time: 5 minutes
Serves: 1
5 Ingredients or Less, 30 Minutes or Less, Keto

The term "bulletproof coffee" comes from the book *The Bulletproof Diet* by Dave Asprey (more on bulletproof coffee on page 63). People have strong opinions about which fats to use, so experiment and decide which ingredients work best for you. If you aren't familiar with ghee, it is clarified butter; it does not have milk solids or milk sugar (lactose). MCT is medium-chain triglyceride and is clear and flavorless, so if you don't like the coconut flavor in your coffee, use MCT. MCT is also better for keeping you in ketosis. Drinking a bulletproof coffee during your fast would be considered a dirty fast.

1 to 2 cups hot coffee

1 teaspoon to
  2 tablespoons MCT or
  coconut oil

1 to 2 tablespoons
  unsalted butter or ghee

Sea salt

Ground cinnamon,
  for seasoning

In a blender, combine the hot coffee, MCT, and butter. Season with salt and cinnamon to taste. Blend until frothy. Alternatively, combine the ingredients in a large bowl and use an immersion blender to combine.

Variation tip: Make bulletproof tea by substituting tea for the coffee. Add a few drops of vanilla extract and a clove for a chai or gingerbread flavor.

Per Serving: Calories: 145; Total Fat: 16g; Total Carbs: <1g; Fiber: 0g; Sugar: 0g; Protein 1g; Sodium: 4mg

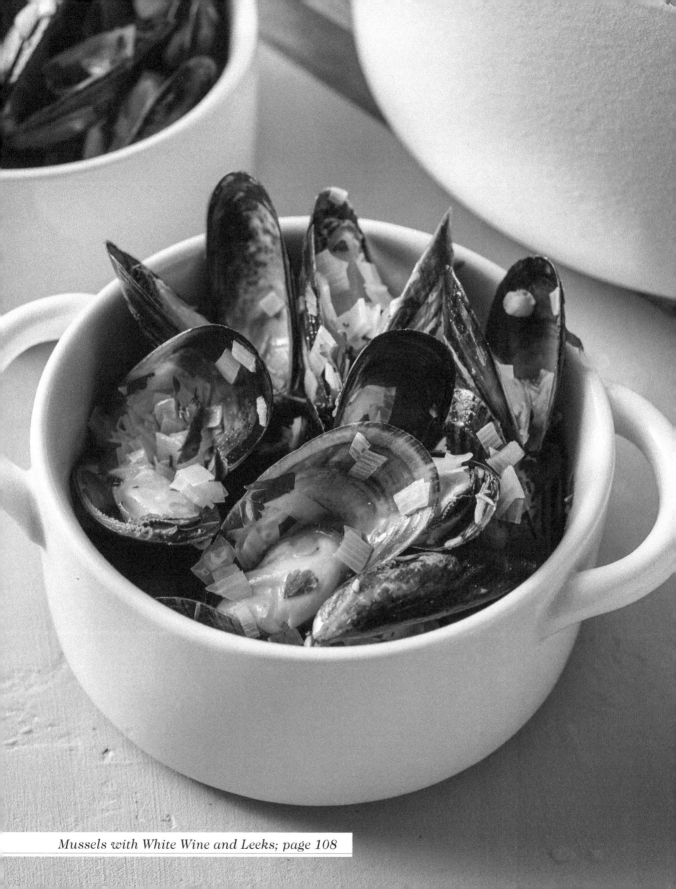

Mussels with White Wine and Leeks; page 108

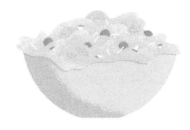

CHAPTER NINE

Low-Carb Recipes

The low-carb, moderate-fat recipes in this chapter are ideal for someone with diabetes. They are similar to keto recipes, but not as high in fat. A classic keto diet will have 4 grams of fat for every 1 gram of carbohydrate and protein combined, and fat really is the dominant nutrient. For these low-carb recipes, I've included fats in typical proportions. If you want keto-specific recipes, you'll find those in chapter 12. If you have diabetes, consult with your doctor before embarking on a specific diet to manage your diabetes and insulin.

Arugula Salad with Tuna

Prep time: 15 minutes
Serves: 1 or 2
30 Minutes or Less, Clean Eating, Low-Carb

Peppery arugula pairs well with the tuna and lemon dressing in this recipe, and olives and capers add a nice saltiness. If you normally eat the entire can of tuna yourself, then consider this a "serves one" recipe.

2 cups baby arugula leaves

1 (5-ounce) can water-packed tuna, drained

1 tomato, diced

1 cup diced cucumber

20 pitted black olives

2 teaspoons capers, drained

2 tablespoons freshly squeezed lemon juice

1 tablespoon extra-virgin olive oil

½ teaspoon dried oregano

Salt

Freshly ground black pepper

1. Place 1 cup of arugula leaves in each of two serving bowls.

2. Place ½ can of tuna on the arugula in each bowl. Evenly divide the tomato, cucumber, olives, and capers between the bowls.

3. In a small bowl, whisk together the lemon juice, oil, oregano, and salt and pepper to taste to blend. Drizzle the dressing over each salad.

Variation tip: Use grilled sardines in place of the tuna.

Per Serving: Calories: 386; Total Fat: 24g; Total Carbs: 19g; Fiber: 6g; Sugar: 7g; Protein 29g; Sodium: 1062mg

Greek Village Salad

Prep time: 15 minutes
Serves: 2
30 Minutes or Less, Clean Eating, Low-Carb

This is my favorite salad recipe, and the not-so-secret ingredient is white wine vinegar, not balsamic. Trust me on this one. My second secret is thinly sliced red onion. I've perfected this to get a paper-thin slice—that way, the onion doesn't overpower the other flavors in the salad.

2 tomatoes, cut into large cubes
2 mini cucumbers, cut into slices
10 paper-thin slices red onion
2 ounces Greek feta cheese
2 tablespoons black Kalamata olives, pitted
1 tablespoon extra-virgin olive oil
1 tablespoon white wine vinegar
¼ teaspoon dried oregano
¼ teaspoon dried basil, or 1 tablespoon finely minced fresh basil leaves
Salt
Freshly ground black pepper

1. In a medium bowl, combine the tomatos, cucumbers, and red onion. Top with the feta cheese and olives.

2. In a small bowl, whisk together the oil, vinegar, oregano, basil, and salt and pepper to taste to blend. Pour the dressing over the salad and gently toss to coat.

3. If you are eating carbs, enjoy this salad with a slice of crusty bread to soak up the dressing.

Variation tip: Try this recipe with avocado in place of the cucumber—it's delicious.

Per Serving: Calories: 207; Total Fat: 15g; Total Carbs: 13g; Fiber: 3g; Sugar: 9g; Protein 6g; Sodium: 612mg

Sour Cream and Onion Egg Salad Lettuce Wraps

Prep time: 25 minutes

Serves: 1

30 Minutes or Less, Low-Carb

My favorite potato chip flavor is sour cream and onion. If you're with me on that, you'll love this recipe. This is such a flavorful, dare I say, decadent egg salad, you won't miss the bread.

2 large hard-boiled
  eggs, peeled
3 tablespoons full-fat
  sour cream
1 tablespoon dried
  onion flakes
2 scallions, finely diced
Salt
Freshly ground
  black pepper
2 to 4 large lettuce leaves
Paprika, for
  seasoning (optional)

1. In a medium bowl, smash the hard-boiled eggs with a fork until lumpy, not smooth.

2. Stir in the sour cream, onion flakes, scallions, and salt and pepper to taste. Spoon the egg salad into the lettuce leaves.

3. Garnish with the paprika (if using).

Variation tip: Make this a curry egg salad lettuce wrap. After smashing the eggs in step 1, stir in 2 tablespoons of mayonnaise, 1 teaspoon of curry powder, and 2 tablespoons of finely chopped celery. Spoon into the lettuce leaves and garnish with fresh cilantro, chives, and paprika, as desired.

Per Serving: Calories: 265; Total Fat: 19g; Total Carbs: 9g; Fiber: 2g; Sugar: 5g; Protein 15g; Sodium: 147mg

Peanut Chicken Lettuce Wraps

Prep time: 10 minutes, plus 20 minutes to marinate / **Cook time:** 15 minutes
Serves: 2 to 4
Low-Carb

This is a fun meal for entertaining. Just increase all the quantities based on the number of guests you're feeding, and rather than assemble the wraps, put the ingredients on the table and let your guests assemble their own. My kids love this meal for this reason.

1 boneless, skinless chicken breast, cut into finger-length strips

½ cup plus 1 tablespoon peanut sauce, divided

8 large lettuce leaves, such as iceberg

1 cup enoki mushrooms (see tip)

½ red bell pepper, thinly sliced

1 (3-inch) piece cucumber, cut into slices

½ cup shredded carrot

6 to 12 cilantro sprigs

6 to 12 fresh mint leaves

1. In a shallow bowl, combine the chicken and ½ cup of peanut sauce. Cover and let marinate at room temperature for 20 minutes.

2. Preheat a grill to medium heat or the oven to 350°F.

3. Remove the chicken from the marinade and place it on the grill. Cook for about 7 minutes per side, until the chicken is cooked through and the juices run clear. Alternatively, place the chicken on a baking sheet and bake for 25 to 30 minutes, until cooked through. Discard the marinade.

4. Place a lettuce leaf on a plate. Add 1 to 3 pieces of chicken, 4 to 9 mushrooms, 1 or 2 red pepper slices, 2 or 3 cucumber slices, 1 tablespoon shredded carrot, 2 or 3 cilantro sprigs, and 2 or 3 mint leaves. Roll up the lettuce leaf, folding in the ends as you roll.

5. Serve the remaining 1 tablespoon of peanut sauce in a small bowl for dipping.

Substitution tip: Use any type of mushroom you like. If you don't mind getting a little more carbs in your diet, use rice paper instead of lettuce leaves. Although the rice paper does have carbs, it's only 11 grams per wrap. You can also use rice noodles as one of your wrap ingredients.

Per Serving: Calories: 256; Total Fat: 8g; Total Carbs: 32g; Fiber: 7g; Sugar: 23g; Protein 18g; Sodium: 56mg

Mediterranean Salad Plate

Prep time: 30 minutes
Serves: 2
30 Minutes or Less, Clean Eating, Low-Carb

I've had many cold plate salads like this in Spain. When served, each ingredient had its own section on the plate, so that's how I describe it here. Although potato is a carb, a boiled potato that's cooled has more resistant starch and, therefore, a lower glycemic and lower insulin response, further reduced by the acid in the lemon juice.

For the salad

1 (5-ounce) can
 water-packed
 tuna, drained
2 to 4 large hard-boiled
 eggs, cooled and peeled
6 new potatoes, boiled
 and chilled
4 ounces green beans,
 steamed and chilled
2 hearts of palm
4 artichoke heart halves
4 thin slices red onion
10 pitted black olives
1 teaspoon capers, drained

For the lemon yogurt dressing

¼ cup plain
 unsweetened yogurt
2 tablespoons extra-virgin
 olive oil
1 tablespoon
 grainy mustard
1 small garlic clove, minced
1 tablespoon freshly
 squeezed lemon juice
½ teaspoon dried oregano
Salt
Freshly ground
 black pepper
1 tablespoon chopped
 fresh parsley

To make the salad

1. In each of two shallow bowls, arrange half the tuna, eggs, potatoes, green beans, hearts of palm, and artichoke hearts. Top with half the red onion, olives, and capers.

To make the lemon yogurt dressing

2. In a small bowl, whisk together the yogurt, oil, mustard, garlic, lemon juice, oregano, and salt and pepper to taste to blend. Divide the dressing between the salads and sprinkle each with fresh parsley.

Make-ahead tip: If you have leftover cooked potatoes, green beans, and hard-boiled eggs or another cold vegetable, this plate comes together in a snap.

Variation tip: To help use up the hearts of palm and artichoke hearts, use them to make a dressing alternative. In a food processor, blend 6 artichoke halves, 1 heart of palm, 2 tablespoons of extra-virgin olive oil, 1 tablespoon of freshly squeezed lemon juice, 1 teaspoon of grainy mustard, and ¼ teaspoon of dried oregano. You'll be able to make the salad plate once and the dressing twice, using all the ingredients without waste.

Per Serving: Calories: 451; Total Fat: 23g; Total Carbs: 40g; Fiber: 8g; Sugar: 8g; Protein 26g; Sodium: 1435mg

Faux Crab Ceviche-Style Salad

Prep time: 20 minutes
Serves: 4 to 8
30 Minutes or Less, Low-Carb, One Pot

This was originally a ceviche recipe using raw fish, which I adapted to use faux crab, and the result is spectacular. All my guests love this recipe, and it's great for entertaining.

1 pound imitation
flake-style crabmeat
½ cup freshly squeezed
lime juice (from about
4 limes)
1 large tomato, chopped
1 tablespoon finely diced
white onion
½ teaspoon finely diced
jalapeño pepper
2 tablespoons minced
fresh cilantro
½ teaspoon salt
1 large avocado,
halved, pitted, peeled,
and cubed
Freshly ground
black pepper

1. In a large bowl, stir together the crabmeat and lime juice to coat well. Stir in the tomato, onion, jalapeño, cilantro, and salt, being careful not to overmix.

2. Add the avocado and mix just to incorporate. Taste and season with pepper as needed.

Serving tip: You can eat this as a seafood salad appetizer, serving 6 to 8, or over lettuce greens to make a meal for up to 4.

Per Serving: Calories: 204; Total Fat: 8g; Total Carbs: 24g; Fiber: 4g; Sugar: 6g; Protein 11g; Sodium: 808mg

Salmon with Mustard, Maple, and Pecans

Prep time: 5 minutes / **Cook time:** 15 minutes
Serves: 2
5 Ingredients or Less, 30 Minutes or Less, Clean Eating, Low-Carb, One Pot

Salmon's high level of omega-3 fatty acids makes it an excellent anti-inflammatory protein. This dish is great served hot, and if there are any leftovers, it tastes great cold the next day.

2 tablespoons grainy mustard
1 tablespoon maple syrup
10 ounces salmon, halved
½ cup pecans, roughly chopped

1. Preheat the oven to 400°F. Line a baking sheet with parchment paper.

2. In a small bowl, stir together the mustard and maple syrup.

3. Place the salmon pieces on the prepared baking sheet. Brush with the maple-mustard sauce and sprinkle with the pecans.

4. Bake for 15 minutes, then check for doneness. There should be no glassy appearance in the fish, and the flesh should flake easily with a fork. Serve with your favorite vegetable, if desired.

Variation tip: This dish is also great with chopped pistachios instead of pecans.

Per Serving: Calories: 392; Total Fat: 26g; Total Carbs: 11g; Fiber: 3g; Sugar: 10g; Protein 31g; Sodium: 573mg

Mussels with White Wine and Leeks

Prep time: 30 minutes / **Cook time:** 15 minutes
Serves: 2 to 4
Clean Eating, Low-Carb, One Pot

If you want an elegant meal on a budget, look no further. I purchased two pounds of mussels at my local fish market for $6—now that's an affordable protein! Although cleaning the mussels is a bit of work, cooking the dish is a snap. Traditionally these mussels would be served with crusty bread used to soak up the broth, but if you're following a low-carb diet, just enjoy this wonderful broth with a spoon after your mussels are finished.

2 pounds mussels

8 cups cold water

2 tablespoons sea salt

1 small leek

1 tablespoon extra-virgin olive oil

1 tablespoon unsalted butter

2 garlic cloves, minced

4 thyme sprigs

1 cup dry white wine

1 tablespoon Bone Broth (page 92; optional)

1 tablespoon chopped fresh parsley

1. Place the mussels in a clean sink full of water. Scrub them with a brush to remove their beards. Rinse and soak again if still gritty. Drain.

2. In a large pot or bowl, combine the mussels, cold water, and salt. Let soak for 10 minutes. Discard any open mussels. Rinse the remaining mussels.

3. Cut the leek lengthwise, remove the greens, and clean well. Chop the white parts medium-fine. Set aside.

4. In a large pot over medium-low heat, heat the oil and melt the butter. Add the chopped leek to the pot and cook for 4 to 6 minutes, until softened.

5. Add the garlic and reduce the heat to low. Remove the thyme leaves from the stems and add them to the pot along with the white wine and bone broth (if using). Increase the heat to medium-high.

6. Add the mussels and cover the pot. Steam for 5 to 7 minutes; if the mussels are open, they're ready. Discard any mussels that don't open. Stir in the fresh parsley. Spoon the mussels and broth into shallow bowls and serve.

Ingredient tip: Holding the stem at one end, slide your thumb and index finger down the thyme sprig and the small leaves will pop off.

Substitution tip: If you don't like leeks, substitute two shallots.

Per Serving: Calories: 632; Total Fat: 23g; Total Carbs: 28g; Fiber: 1g; Sugar: 3g; Protein 55g; Sodium: 1315mg

Caramelized Onion and Mushroom Soup

Prep time: 15 minutes / **Cook time:** 40 minutes
Serves: 4
Clean Eating, Low-Carb, One Pot

I used dried mushrooms here as they're more shelf stable; they're a good pantry item that can store for a long time. Dried mushrooms can also have a deeper flavor than fresh, and using the mushroom-soaking liquid adds even more depth of flavor to this tasty soup. When you use the mushroom-soaking liquid, be careful not to use any of the sediment that will fall to the bottom of the bowl.

½ cup dried mushrooms
2 cups boiling water
1 tablespoon extra-virgin
  olive oil
6 small yellow onions,
  quartered and cut
  into slices
1¼ teaspoons salt, divided
2 teaspoons butter
¼ cup dry white wine
  or vermouth
2 garlic cloves, crushed
½ teaspoon thyme
4 cups no-sodium
  vegetable, chicken,
  or beef broth
Freshly ground
  black pepper
1 teaspoon grated
  Parmesan cheese

1. Break the dried mushrooms into small pieces and discard any hard stems. Place the pieces into a heatproof bowl. Pour in the boiling water and let soak for about 10 minutes, until softened.

2. In a large pot over medium-low heat, heat the oil.

3. Add the onions and ½ teaspoon of salt. Cook for 5 to 7 minutes, until softened. Increase the heat to medium-high and add the butter.

4. Let the onions cook for 2 to 3 minutes more, until browned, then add 2 tablespoons of wine to deglaze the pot, scraping up any browned bits from the bottom. When the mixture gets dry, add 2 tablespoons more of the wine and continue to deglaze the pot. Continue this process, cooking for about 10 minutes more, until the onions are a caramel color and all the wine has been added. If you need more liquid, use small amounts of the mushroom soaking liquid or broth.

5. Stir in the garlic, mushrooms, mushroom soaking liquid, and thyme. Add the broth and remaining ¾ teaspoon of salt. Bring to a simmer and cook for 10 minutes.

6. Spoon into four bowls, season with pepper to taste, and divide the Parmesan cheese among the bowls.

Variation tip: Make this in the style of French onion soup. Transfer this soup into a heatproof bowl, add a slice of dried bread, and top with a slice of Emmental, mozzarella, or Swiss cheese. Broil, watching closely, until the cheese melts. If you want a clear broth to enjoy as part of your fast, strain out the onions and mushrooms.

Per Serving: Calories: 149; Total Fat: 6g; Total Carbs: 20g; Fiber: 3g; Sugar: 7g; Protein 3g; Sodium: 791mg

Low-Carb Buffalo Chicken Casserole

Prep time: 15 minutes / **Cook time:** 25 minutes
Serves: 4
Low-Carb, One Pot

I love the flavor of buffalo chicken wings but hate the mess. This recipe will remind you of the flavor of buffalo wings, but it uses two parts cauliflower for every one part chicken.

½ cup cream cheese, at
  room temperature
⅓ cup chopped scallions
¼ cup buffalo wing sauce
¼ cup blue cheese
  salad dressing
4 cups grated cauliflower
2 cups cubed
  cooked chicken
½ cup grated Emmental
  cheese or cheese
  of choice
Paprika, for seasoning

1. Preheat the oven to 400°F.

2. In a medium bowl, stir together the cream cheese, scallions, buffalo wing sauce, and blue cheese dressing.

3. Add the grated cauliflower and cooked chicken and toss to combine and coat. Pour the mixture into a 9-by-11-inch casserole dish. Sprinkle with the Emmental cheese.

4. Bake for 25 minutes, until hot and bubbly. Sprinkle with the paprika before serving.

Variation tip: If full-fat cream cheese is too much fat for you to tolerate, use a lower-fat version.

Per Serving: Calories: 325; Total Fat: 22g; Total Carbs: 9g; Fiber: 2g; Sugar: 5g; Protein 24g; Sodium: 1129mg

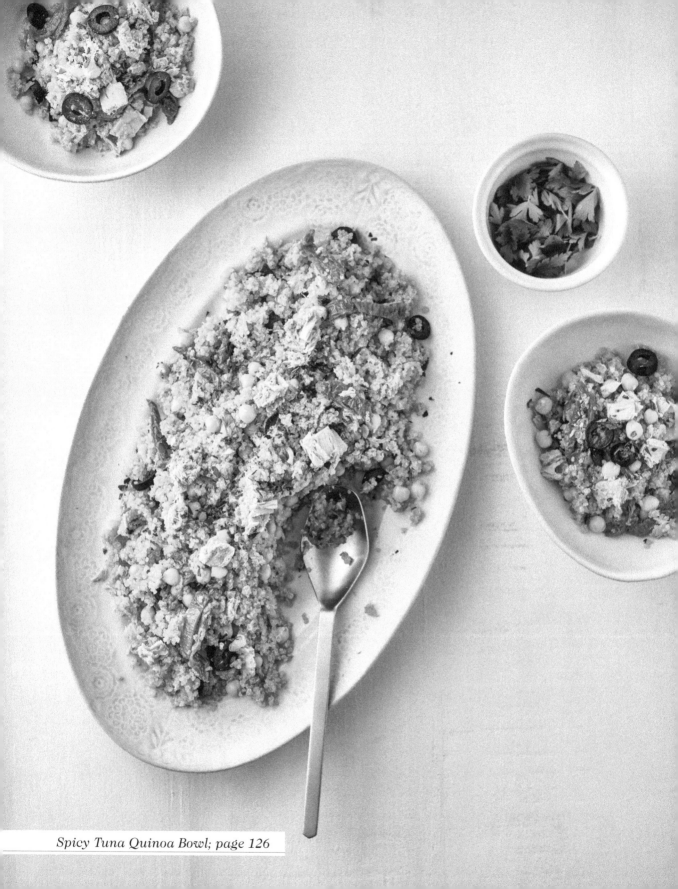

Spicy Tuna Quinoa Bowl; page 126

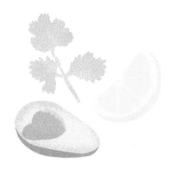

CHAPTER TEN

Low-Calorie/Low-Fat Recipes

This section is intended for those who can't tolerate high amounts of fat or for your modified fasting day, as all these recipes are under 400 calories. These recipes are also perfect if you can't tolerate the high-fat requirements of keto or other diabetic diets. I've included an assortment of breakfasts, lunches, and dinners.

Overnight Rolled Oats with Cinnamon

Prep time: 10 minutes, plus overnight to rest
Serves: 4
5 Ingredients or Less, Clean Eating, Low-Calorie, Low-Fat

One issue intermittent fasters can have is getting enough fiber to keep their digestive system regular. Breaking your fast with a good source of soluble fiber can be just what you need to keep your digestive system happy. Soluble fiber also provides a slow rise in blood sugar. Because these oats are made the night before, you'll have zero prep when you're ready to break your fast, and you can enjoy them as your "break-fast" whatever the time of day.

¾ cup yogurt

½ cup old-fashioned rolled oats

1 teaspoon maple syrup

¼ teaspoon ground cinnamon

Pinch salt (optional)

Fresh berries, for serving (optional)

1 banana, cut into slices (optional)

Nuts, for serving (optional)

Seeds, for serving (optional)

In a lidded container, stir together the yogurt, oats, syrup, cinnamon, and salt (if using) to blend. Cover and refrigerate overnight. Serve with your favorite toppings, as desired.

Variation tip: Even old-fashioned or "10-minute oats" can be quickly prepared in the microwave. In a small microwave-safe bowl, combine ½ cup of oats with 1 cup of water, milk, or plant-based milk (or half water and half milk). Microwave for 1 to 2 minutes. Stir in the cinnamon, maple syrup, and 2 tablespoons of yogurt, along with your favorite toppings.

Per Serving: Calories: 72; Total Fat: 1g; Total Carbs: 11g; Fiber: 1g; Sugar: 4g; Protein 4g; Sodium: 33mg

Cherry-Almond Chia

Prep time: 10 minutes, plus overnight to rest
Serves: 1
5 Ingredients or Less, Clean Eating, Low-Calorie, Low-Fat

If you had a chia pet as a kid, you know all about chia seeds. But instead of sprouting them on a clay pet, you'll soak these seeds in yogurt overnight. These water-loving seeds absorb up to twelve times their weight in liquid to form a gel. Chia is a complete protein and an abundant plant source of omega-3s. In a study that compared plain yogurt to yogurt plus chia as a morning snack, yogurt plus chia resulted in better satiety, reduced hunger, and eating a smaller lunch.

¾ cup plain yogurt

2 tablespoons chia seeds

½ teaspoon almond extract

2 tablespoons dried
  sour cherries

2 tablespoons almonds,
  chopped and toasted

In a lidded container, stir together the yogurt, chia seeds, and almond extract. Cover and refrigerate overnight. The next morning, add the dried cherries and toasted almonds.

Variation tip: Make this recipe your own by choosing other fruit and nut combinations, such as dried apricot and pistachio or dried cranberry and toasted walnut.

Per Serving: Calories: 399; Total Fat: 18g; Total Carbs: 44g;
Fiber: 13g; Sugar: 27g; Protein 17g; Sodium: 131mg

Lemon-Lavender Muffins

Prep time: 20 minutes / **Cook time:** 16 minutes
Makes: 12 small muffins
Clean Eating, Low-Fat

With no butter or oil and only one egg, these low-fat muffins are still full of flavor, thanks to the lemon and complementary lavender flavor. Although we often associate lavender with soap, perfume, and aromatherapy, culinary-grade lavender buds are edible and they add a mild floral bouquet to the muffins.

For the muffins

⅔ cup granulated sugar
2 teaspoons culinary-grade
  lavender buds
2 cups barley flour or
  all-purpose flour
1 teaspoon baking powder
½ teaspoon salt
1 large egg
3 tablespoons freshly
  squeezed lemon juice
1 tablespoon lemon pulp
1 teaspoon grated
  lemon zest
⅔ cup plus 2 tablespoons
  soy milk
½ cup unsweetened
  applesauce

For the glaze (optional)

½ cup confectioners' sugar
1 tablespoon freshly
  squeezed lemon juice
2 teaspoons grated lemon
  zest, divided

To make the muffins

1. Preheat the oven to 375°F. Line the cups of a standard muffin tin with paper liners.

2. In a food processor, blend the granulated sugar and lavender buds for 3 to 4 minutes. Strain the mixture through a fine-mesh sieve into a bowl. If making the glaze, reserve any larger buds for garnish.

3. In a large bowl, whisk the barley flour, baking powder, and salt to combine. Set aside.

4. Add the egg to the lavender sugar. Using a handheld mixer, blend on low speed for about 3 minutes, until fluffy. Stir in the lemon juice, lemon pulp, lemon zest, soy milk, and applesauce.

5. Add the wet ingredients to the dry ingredients and stir to incorporate. Evenly distribute the batter into the prepared muffin tin.

6. Bake for 14 to 16 minutes, or until a toothpick inserted into the center of a muffin comes out clean. Let the muffins cool until warm.

7. In a small bowl, stir together the confectioners' sugar, lemon juice, and 1 teaspoon of lemon zest. Top each muffin with 1 teaspoon of glaze (if using).

8. Sprinkle the muffins with the remaining 1 teaspoon of zest and garnish with the reserved lavender buds.

9. Refrigerate leftovers in an airtight container for up to 3 days.

Variation tip: You can also make a lime version. Just swap the lemons for an equal amount of lime juice, pulp, and zest.

Per Serving (1 muffin): Calories: 129; Total Fat: 1g; Total Carbs: 29g; Fiber: 4g; Sugar: 13g; Protein 3g; Sodium: 154mg

Easy Tofu Scramble

Prep time: 5 minutes / **Cook time:** 10 minutes
Serves: 2 to 4
30 Minutes or Less, Clean Eating, Low-Calorie, Low-Fat, One Pot

This has got to be one of the easiest recipes in this collection. It's low-fat, high in protein, and packed with great flavor. Tofu is made from soybeans, a complete protein. This scramble has 23 grams of protein per serving and both essential fatty acids—omega-6 and omega-3.

1 teaspoon extra-virgin
   olive oil
1 pound firm tofu
⅛ teaspoon
   ground turmeric
1 tablespoon nutritional
   yeast flakes, plus more
   as needed
½ teaspoon salt, plus more
   as needed
⅛ teaspoon garlic powder,
   plus more as needed
Freshly ground
   black pepper

1. In a nonstick skillet over medium heat, heat the oil.

2. Roughly crumble the tofu with your hands (not too finely) and add it to the heated pan. Stir the tofu to coat with the oil.

3. Sprinkle in the turmeric and stir to get a consistent pale-yellow color throughout.

4. Stir in the nutritional yeast, salt, and garlic powder to incorporate. Taste and adjust the seasonings to suit. Add the pepper to taste.

5. Serve as you would scrambled eggs, with a side of salsa, sliced tomato, avocado, and/or toast, as desired.

Variation tip: This dish is vegan and low-fat, but you can add pieces of sausage to your scramble, if you like.

Substitution tip: Rather than garlic powder, sauté 1 tablespoon of chopped onion and 1 garlic clove, minced, in the oil until softened before you add the tofu.

Per Serving: Calories: 249; Total Fat: 13g; Total Carbs: 7g; Fiber: 2g; Sugar: 1g; Protein 23g; Sodium: 610mg

Low-Fat Sicilian Eggs

Prep time: 10 minutes / **Cook time:** 15 minutes

Serves: 2

30 Minutes or Less, Clean Eating, Low-Carb, Low-Fat, One Pot

My grandmother used to make eggs this way. My dad taught me and I taught my daughter, and she says this is her favorite recipe in the book. This is the low-fat version of my grandmother's recipe. Mediterranean cooking has many benefits, including those from the use of tomato sauces, olive oil, and herbs and spices.

1 teaspoon extra-virgin olive oil

⅓ cup chopped Spanish onion or white onion

1 (14.5-ounce) diced tomatoes, with juices, blended with an immersion blender

1 teaspoon sugar (optional)

⅛ teaspoon salt

4 large eggs

2 tablespoons finely minced fresh basil leaves

1 teaspoon grated low-fat Parmesan cheese

1. In a skillet over medium heat, heat the oil.

2. Add the onion and cook for 4 to 6 minutes, stirring occasionally, until soft.

3. Add the blended tomatoes and increase the heat to medium-high to get the tomatoes bubbling. Taste and add the sugar (if using) and salt.

4. Crack the eggs into the hot tomato mixture. If you want your eggs cooked on top (as opposed to sunny-side up), reduce the heat and partially cover the skillet, leaving room for steam to escape. Cook for 2 to 3 minutes. Add the basil. Cook for 1 to 2 minutes more, or until the eggs are cooked the way you prefer. You can also scramble your eggs in the tomato sauce, if you like.

5. Top with the grated Parmesan cheese.

Variation tip: To make homemade tomato sauce: Boil water in a large pot. Using a slotted spoon, lower 6 ripe Roma tomatoes, a few at a time, into the boiling water. Boil for about 3 minutes, or until the skin cracks. Pour the hot tomatoes into a colander and rinse with cold water. Cut the cores from the tomatoes and squeeze the tomato (the skin will come off) into a food processor. Process until mostly smooth. Transfer the tomatoes to the pot and add ½ teaspoon of salt and 2 teaspoons of sugar.

Per Serving: Calories: 240; Total Fat: 13g; Total Carbs: 15g; Fiber: 4g; Sugar: 10g; Protein 15g; Sodium: 229mg

Kale Salad with Roasted Sweet Potato, Pepitas, and Raspberry Vinaigrette

Prep time: 20 minutes / **Cook time:** 30 minutes
Serves: 2 to 4
Clean Eating, Low-Calorie, Low-Fat

Between the bitter kale, sweet potatoes, and tangy vinaigrette, this recipe's got it all. All except fat, that is, as we keep the added fat and oils low here. Although, the toasted pumpkin seeds do add a bit of healthy fat, as well as some flavorful crunch. For added protein, serve this salad with grilled seasoned chicken breast or cubed tofu.

For the salad

- 1 sweet potato, peeled and cubed
- 1 tablespoon extra-virgin olive oil
- 1 teaspoon dried rosemary leaves, crumbled
- ⅛ teaspoon salt
- ⅛ teaspoon freshly ground black pepper
- 1 bunch kale, chopped (4 cups)
- 2 tablespoons pumpkin seeds, toasted
- 2 tablespoons dried cranberries

To make the salad

1. Preheat the oven to 400°F. Line a baking sheet with parchment paper.

2. In a medium bowl, stir together the sweet potato, oil, rosemary, salt, and pepper until the potato is coated. Transfer to the prepared baking sheet in a single layer.

3. Roast for 15 minutes. Turn the sweet potato and cook for 15 minutes more, or until fork-tender.

4. Put the kale in a large bowl. Top with the roasted sweet potato, toasted pumpkin seeds, and cranberries.

To make the dressing

5. In a blender, puree the raspberries. Press the puree through a fine-mesh sieve set over a bowl to remove the seeds. Stir the yogurt, maple syrup, and vinegar into the strained puree. Drizzle the dressing over the salad and enjoy.

Variation tip: Here are some salad combinations that go well with kale to create a delicious salad:

- Apple, walnuts, and blue cheese
- Beets, walnuts, and goat cheese
- Pomegranate seeds and roasted tofu
- Sliced almonds and Brussels sprouts

Per Serving: Calories: 281; Total Fat: 12g; Total Carbs: 42g; Fiber: 9g; Sugar: 22g; Protein 6g; Sodium: 151mg

For the dressing

1 cup raspberries, fresh or frozen

2 tablespoons low-fat or fat-free plain yogurt

4 teaspoons maple syrup

2 teaspoons white wine vinegar

Umami Lentil Patties

Prep time: 25 minutes / **Cook time:** 30 minutes
Serves: 4
Clean Eating, Low-Fat

I make my veggie patties with lentils because I don't need to soak them ahead and I can cook the patties in about 15 minutes. There was a diet book that advised against eating lentils and other legumes as they are high in lectins (also called "anti-nutrients"), but lectins are removed from beans, peas, and lentils with cooking.

1 cup dried lentils
  (red, green, or brown)
4 cups water, plus more
  as needed
5 dried shiitake mushrooms
1 cup boiling water
¼ cup nutritional yeast
2 tablespoons
  chopped walnuts
2 tablespoons
  ground flaxseed
½ teaspoon salt, plus more
  as needed
Freshly ground
  black pepper
2 tablespoons bread
  crumbs (optional)
1 teaspoon extra-virgin
  olive oil

1. In a large pot over high heat, combine the lentils and enough water to cover by 1 inch. Cover the pot and bring to a boil. Reduce the heat to maintain a simmer and cook the lentils for 15 minutes, until soft but not mushy (red lentils cook to a softer texture than brown or green).

2. While the lentils cook, in a small bowl, combine the mushrooms and boiling water. Let sit to soften.

3. Drain the lentils and let sit for about 5 minutes. Pour half the lentils into a bowl and puree using an immersion blender, or add to a regular blender and puree and return to the pot. Add the remaining whole lentils.

4. Remove the mushrooms from the water and cut them into small pieces. Reserve the soaking water.

5. Stir the mushrooms, nutritional yeast, walnuts, flaxseed, and salt into the lentils. Taste and add more salt, as needed, and pepper to taste. Form the mixture into 4 patties; if it's too wet and sticky, stir in the bread crumbs so the patties stick together. If the mixture is too dry, use some of the soaking liquid from the mushrooms to moisten it.

6. In a nonstick skillet over medium-high heat, heat the oil and swirl to coat the skillet.

7. Working in batches, if needed, place the patties in the hot skillet. Reshape slightly, if needed, but resist the temptation to press the patty into the pan. Cook for about 7 minutes; don't flip too soon or the patty could come apart. Flip and cook the opposite side for about 7 minutes more, until browned on each side and the patties hold together when flipped.

8. Serve on a bun, if you like, but because the lentils are starchy, I prefer them without. Alternatively, shape the lentil mixture into rounds and make meatless meatballs.

Make-ahead tip: Prepare the patties and refrigerate them in an airtight container for up to 48 hours, or freeze for up to 1 month. Proceed with step 6 to cook.

Variation tip: To grill, refrigerate or freeze the patties for at least 4 hours. Spray with nonstick spray and place on a hot grill over indirect heat. Cook for 5 to 8 minutes before gently flipping and cooking the other side for 5 to 8 minutes more.

Per Serving: Calories: 264; Total Fat: 6g; Total Carbs: 38g; Fiber: 9g; Sugar: 1g; Protein 18g; Sodium: 302mg

Spicy Tuna Quinoa Bowl

Prep time: 15 minutes / **Cook time:** 25 minutes
Serves: 4
Clean Eating, Low-Fat, One Pot

Quinoa has all the essential amino acids our bodies need, making it a complete protein. In fact, this dish gets protein from three sources: quinoa, chickpeas, and tuna. This dish delivers great textures from the quinoa and chickpeas, a lively kick from the red pepper flakes, and a salty burst of flavor from the olives and sun-dried tomatoes. Other than the fresh parsley garnish, this is a total pantry recipe.

1 onion, chopped

4 cups unsalted vegetable broth, divided

2 garlic cloves, minced

½ teaspoon red pepper flakes

¾ cup quinoa, rinsed

1 (5-ounce) can water-packed tuna, drained

1 (15.5-ounce) can chickpeas, drained and rinsed

½ cup sliced black olives

½ cup oil-packed sun-dried tomatoes, sliced

¼ teaspoon salt

1 tablespoon chopped fresh parsley

1. In a medium pot over medium heat, combine the onion and 1 to 2 tablespoons of vegetable broth. Cook for about 5 minutes, until soft.

2. Add the garlic and red pepper flakes and reduce the heat to medium-low. Add 1 to 2 more tablespoons of broth if the mixture is dry. Cook, stirring, for about 3 minutes, or until the garlic is softened.

3. Add the remaining vegetable broth and quinoa. Increase the heat to high and bring the mixture to a boil. Reduce the heat to maintain a simmer and cook for 15 minutes, until the quinoa opens. Turn off the heat but keep the pot on the stove.

4. Stir in the tuna, chickpeas, olives, and sun-dried tomatoes to incorporate. Let sit for 10 to 15 minutes, or until the liquid is mostly absorbed. Taste and season with salt as desired. Serve in shallow bowls topped with fresh parsley.

Addition tip: To make this a more balanced meal, enjoy with a side of steamed vegetables.

Per Serving: Calories: 307; Total Fat: 6g; Total Carbs: 47g; Fiber: 9g; Sugar: 10g; Protein 18g; Sodium: 526mg

Garlic Shrimp

Prep time: 10 minutes, plus 10 minutes to marinate / **Cook time:** 6 minutes
Serves: 4
5 Ingredients or Less, 30 Minutes or Less, Clean Eating, Low-Carb, Low-Fat, One Pot

The secret to getting the shrimp to cook properly is buying them raw but deveined and cut down the back, sometimes sold frozen as E-Z peel shrimp. Don't use pre-cooked or peeled shrimp for this, as they'll be too dry. If your shrimp are raw but not deveined, just cut them down the back with kitchen scissors, remove the vein, and leave the shell on. Serve with potato salad or other summer salads to make a complete meal.

1 pound raw deveined
   shrimp, shell on
1 tablespoon extra-virgin
   olive oil
4 garlic cloves, crushed

1. Rinse the shrimp and place in a strainer to remove excess water. Transfer to a medium bowl and add the oil. Stir to coat. Add the garlic and stir to coat. Let the shrimp marinate for 10 minutes, or cover and refrigerate for a couple of hours.

2. Heat a skillet over medium-high heat. Place the shrimp in the skillet, spreading them in a single layer. Cook for 3 minutes, or until the shrimp turn pink. Turn the shrimp and cook the other side for 3 minutes, or until pink. The shrimp will expand and separate from their shells.

Variation tip: These shrimp taste amazing on the grill. For this method, preheat the grill, then turn the heat to medium. Cook the shrimp with the lid closed for 3 minutes per side. Be careful placing the shrimp on the grill so they don't fall between the slats.

Per Serving: Calories: 174; Total Fat: 5g; Total Carbs: 3g; Fiber: <1g; Sugar: 0g; Protein 28g; Sodium: 1071mg

Seared White Fish with Pan-Fried Vegetables

Prep time: 15 minutes / **Cook time:** 15 minutes
Serves: 2
30 Minutes or Less, Clean Eating, Low-Calorie, Low-Carb, Low-Fat

This is the ultimate clean eating recipe. The flavors of this dish are subtle, delicate, and light. You'll feel satisfied but clean after enjoying this fresh summery meal. Add some fresh dill on top, if you have it.

2 teaspoons extra-virgin olive oil or high-oleic sunflower, safflower, or canola oil, divided

1 small onion, finely diced (about ½ cup)

1 carrot, finely diced (about ½ cup)

1 Roma tomato, finely diced (about ½ cup)

1 celery stalk, finely diced (about ¼ cup)

Salt

Freshly ground black pepper

1 pound halibut, cod, or other firm white fish

Fresh dill, for garnish (optional)

1. In a skillet over medium-high heat, heat 1 teaspoon of oil and swirl to coat the skillet.

2. Add the onion, carrot, tomato, and celery. Season with salt and pepper to taste. Cook for 10 to 12 minutes, until the vegetables are soft and juices are present.

3. In a second skillet over medium-high heat, heat the remaining 1 teaspoon of oil and swirl to coat the skillet.

4. Rinse the fish and pat it dry. Season the fish all over with salt and pepper and place the fish in the skillet. Let the fish sear for about 5 minutes. Flip the fish and sear the other side for about 5 minutes. Check that the fish is cooked through. It will no longer appear glassy and the flesh will flake easily with a fork.

5. Plate the fish and top with the pan-fried vegetables. Garnish with fresh dill (if using).

Addition tip: If you're enjoying carbs, this fish pairs well with boiled new potatoes topped with salt, pepper, butter, and fresh dill.

Per Serving: Calories: 288; Total Fat: 8g; Total Carbs: 10g; Fiber: 2g; Sugar: 5g; Protein 43g; Sodium: 195mg

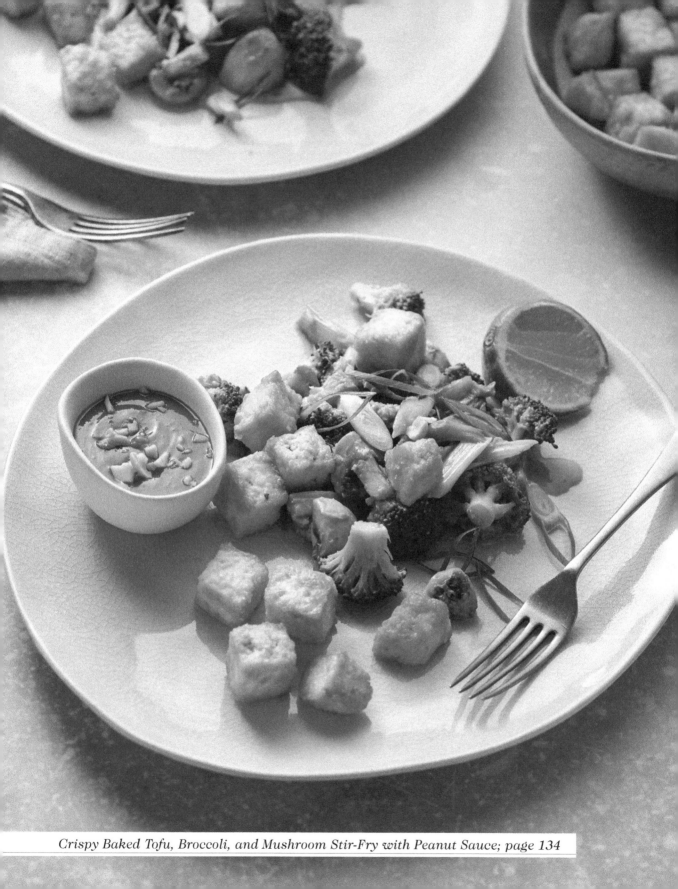

Crispy Baked Tofu, Broccoli, and Mushroom Stir-Fry with Peanut Sauce; page 134

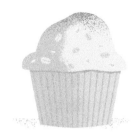

CHAPTER ELEVEN

Clean Eating Recipes

The recipes in this chapter are for general wellness, especially if you want to feel nourished when you break your fast. For clean eating recipes, I don't use any ultra-processed food ingredients. When you break your fast, it's important to be mindful about what you eat. When fasting, you have fewer eating opportunities to nourish your body, so nutrient-rich foods are your best bet. I've included a variety of delicious breakfast, lunch, dinner, and snack options.

Oatmeal Nut Muffins

Prep time: 15 minutes / **Cook time:** 18 minutes
Makes: 12 large muffins
Clean Eating

I use barley flour for baking for a few reasons. Barley flour is a whole-grain flour and an easy substitute for white flour in baking. It's also high in beta-glucan, a fiber that's beneficial for the immune system. The barley flour doesn't brown as much as all-purpose when you cook, so don't go by the color of the muffins to check for doneness—although, because of the maple syrup, these do have a beautiful finished color!

1½ cups barley flour

1 cup old-fashioned rolled oats

2 teaspoons ground cinnamon

1 teaspoon baking powder

½ teaspoon salt

¾ cup dark maple syrup

½ cup high-oleic sunflower oil, safflower oil, or canola oil

½ cup unsweetened soy milk or your favorite milk

2 large eggs

1 cup chopped nuts (see tip)

½ cup unsweetened shredded coconut

1. Preheat the oven to 375°F. Line a 12-cup muffin tin with paper liners and set aside.

2. In a large bowl, stir together the flour, oats, cinnamon, baking powder, and salt. Set aside.

3. In a medium bowl, combine the maple syrup, oil, milk, and eggs. Using a handheld mixer, blend on low speed until combined. Pour the wet ingredients into the dry ingredients and stir to incorporate evenly. Stir in the nuts and coconut to distribute evenly. Scoop the mixture into the prepared muffin tins.

4. Bake for 15 to 18 minutes, or until a toothpick inserted into the center of a muffin comes out clean.

Variation tip: Use whatever nut or combination of nuts you like best. You could also add your favorite dried fruit.

Per Serving (1 muffin): Calories: 311; Total Fat: 19g; Total Carbs: 33g; Fiber: 5g; Sugar: 14g; Protein 6g; Sodium: 158mg

Slow Cooker Coconut Millet with Toasted Coconut and Pistachios

Prep time: 15 minutes / **Cook time:** 2 hours
Serves: 2
Clean Eating, One Pot

I can't tell you how much I like this recipe. I prefer to do it in my small slow cooker rather than stand over the stove, and I also think it tastes better. But no matter how you cook this, I think it will win you over.

⅓ cup millet

2 tablespoons unsweetened shredded coconut

½ (14-ounce) can coconut milk, well shaken

½ cup water

1 tablespoon coconut palm sugar

⅛ teaspoon salt, plus more as needed

1 to 2 tablespoons shredded or shaved coconut, toasted (optional)

1 tablespoon pistachios, toasted (optional)

1. Preheat the slow cooker.

2. In a dry skillet over medium-high heat, toast the millet and the unsweetened coconut for 5 to 7 minutes, stirring or shaking often to prevent burning. When you smell the coconut and the colors get darker, transfer to the slow cooker.

3. Add the coconut milk, water, coconut palm sugar, and salt to the slow cooker and stir.

4. Cover the cooker and cook on low heat for 2 hours. Taste and season with more salt as needed.

5. Serve topped with the toasted coconut (if using) and pistachios (if using) or with your favorite dried or fresh fruit, nuts, or seeds.

Variation tip: You can prepare this on the stovetop. Toast the millet and coconut in a medium pot over medium heat, being careful not to burn them. Add the coconut milk, water, coconut palm sugar, and salt and bring to a simmer, stirring constantly. Cook for 30 minutes, stirring constantly. Turn off the heat, cover, and let sit for 10 minutes, adding more water if needed. Serve topped as desired.

Per Serving: Calories: 348; Total Fat: 22g; Total Carbs: 36g; Fiber: 4g; Sugar: 11g; Protein 5g; Sodium: 102mg

Crispy Baked Tofu, Broccoli, and Mushroom Stir-Fry with Peanut Sauce

Prep time: 20 minutes / **Cook time:** 35 minutes
Serves: 4
Clean Eating

My kids love crispy baked tofu. When I make this recipe, I prepare twice as much as I would for other recipes, as the kids gobble it up. The next time I'm invited to an event that serves cocktails and appetizers, I'll bring these—they're a great little appetizer on their own, even without the stir-fry.

For the baked tofu

- 2 tablespoons low-sodium or regular tamari
- 1½ teaspoons extra-virgin olive oil
- 1 teaspoon garlic powder
- 1 pound firm or extra-firm tofu, cubed
- 1½ tablespoons cornstarch

For the peanut sauce

- ¼ cup peanut butter
- ¼ cup water
- 1½ teaspoons soy sauce
- 1 teaspoon honey
- 1 teaspoon freshly squeezed lime juice
- ⅛ teaspoon red pepper flakes

For the stir-fry

- 1 tablespoon high-oleic sunflower oil, safflower oil, or canola oil
- 1 bunch scallions, cut on the diagonal into 1-inch slices
- 1 or 2 garlic cloves, minced
- 1 (½-inch) piece fresh ginger, peeled and grated
- 4 cups broccoli florets
- 2 cups mushrooms, quartered

To make the baked tofu

1. Preheat the oven to 400°F. Line a baking sheet with parchment paper.

2. In a small bowl, stir together the tamari, oil, and garlic powder. Place the tofu in a shallow bowl and pour the sauce over it. Stir to coat. Let sit for 5 to 10 minutes to absorb the liquid.

3. Sprinkle the tofu with the cornstarch and stir to coat. Evenly distribute the bowl's contents onto the prepared baking sheet.

4. Bake for 10 minutes, flip the tofu, and bake for 10 minutes more, until browned and crispy on the outside.

To make the peanut sauce

5. While the tofu bakes, in a small bowl, whisk together the peanut butter, water, soy sauce, honey, lime juice, and red pepper flakes until smooth. Set aside.

CONTINUED

To make the stir-fry

6. In a large pan over medium heat, heat the oil. Add the scallions, garlic, and ginger. Cook for 2 to 3 minutes, being careful that the garlic does not burn.

7. Add the broccoli and mushrooms. Increase the heat to high and cook for about 3 minutes, stirring constantly.

8. Reduce the heat to medium, add water, 2 tablespoons at a time, if the pan is dry, and cover the pan. Cook for 3 to 4 minutes and check the broccoli for doneness. When the broccoli is almost done, stir in the peanut sauce to coat. Serve with the baked tofu.

Variation tip: Serve with brown rice, quinoa, or cauliflower rice.

Substitution tip: Use almond butter instead of peanut butter.

Per Serving: Calories: 313; Total Fat: 19g; Total Carbs: 19g; Fiber: 5g; Sugar: 6g; Protein 19g; Sodium: 493mg

Corn and Edamame Salad with Ginger Dressing

Prep time: 10 minutes / **Cook time:** 10 minutes
Serves: 4
30 Minutes or Less, Clean Eating, Low-Fat

Edamame are generally sold frozen, either in the shell or loose. They take only 3 minutes to prepare and are great on their own as a snack with a little salt or soy sauce. Like other forms of soy, they have benefits for heart heath, immune function, and cancer protection.

For the dressing

1 tablespoon freshly squeezed lime juice
1 tablespoon low-sodium tamari
1 tablespoon rice vinegar
1 teaspoon high-oleic sunflower oil, safflower oil, or canola oil
1½ teaspoons minced peeled fresh ginger
1 garlic clove, minced

For the salad

2 cups shelled frozen edamame
1 cup fresh or frozen corn
4 scallions, thinly sliced
1 sheet nori seaweed, crumbled

To make the dressing

In a small bowl, whisk together the lime juice, tamari, vinegar, oil, ginger, and garlic to blend. Set aside.

To make the salad

1. Bring a medium pot of water to a boil over high heat. Add the frozen edamame and corn and boil for 3 minutes. Drain. Transfer the edamame and corn to a serving bowl and add the scallions.

2. Add the dressing and toss to coat.

3. Top with crumbled nori.

Craving tip: The strong ginger and tamari flavors here will help bust a craving and leave your mouth refreshed.

Per Serving: Calories: 143; Total Fat: 4g; Total Carbs: 15g; Fiber: 4g; Sugar: 3g; Protein 12g; Sodium: 213mg

Broccoli Slaw with Cranberries and Pistachios

Prep time: 20 minutes, plus 10 minutes to rest
Serves: 4
30 Minutes or Less, Clean Eating

This tasty and colorful slaw calls for broccoli stems, which are often overlooked in favor of the florets. Whenever I make steamed broccoli for my family, I save the stems just for this purpose.

4 or 5 broccoli stems
¼ cup plain
   probiotic yogurt
¼ cup mayonnaise
Juice of 1 lime
Salt
Freshly ground
   black pepper
Cayenne pepper (optional)
¼ cup dried cranberries
¼ cup shelled pistachios

1. Cut away the outer thick parts of the broccoli stems, then process the stems on the shredder setting of a food processor.

2. In a small bowl, stir together the yogurt, mayonnaise, and lime juice. Taste and season with the salt, black pepper, and cayenne (if using).

3. In a large bowl, gently stir together the shredded broccoli stems, dressing, cranberries, and pistachios. Let sit for 10 minutes before serving.

Variation tip: Mix some Brussels sprouts with your broccoli stems.

Per Serving: Calories: 183; Total Fat: 14g; Total Carbs: 13g; Fiber: 2g; Sugar: 9g; Protein 3g; Sodium: 145mg

Lentil and Sweet Potato Tacos with Fresh Guacamole and Pico de Gallo

Prep time: 20 minutes / **Cook time:** 25 minutes
Serves: 4
Clean Eating

This is a great meal for Meatless Monday with the family. Everything is the same as a taco meal, except you use lentils and sweet potato in place of meat. I've made this dish with just lentils, but the sweet potato adds a nice flavor and texture.

For the tacos

1 cup lentils, rinsed

2 cups water

1 small to medium sweet potato, peeled and cut into ½-inch cubes

2 teaspoons extra-virgin olive oil or preferred cooking oil

1 tablespoon taco seasoning, plus more as needed

8 (6-inch) taco shells or (8-inch) soft tortillas

¾ cup shredded sharp Cheddar cheese or other cheese of choice

½ cup sour cream

For the guacamole

1 tablespoon finely diced onion

1 tablespoon fresh cilantro

1½ teaspoons freshly squeezed lime juice

1 teaspoon finely diced jalapeño pepper

⅛ teaspoon salt

1 avocado, halved, pitted, and peeled

For the pico de gallo

1 tomato, finely diced

1 tablespoon finely diced onion

1 tablespoon finely minced fresh cilantro

1 teaspoon finely diced jalapeño pepper

Salt

CONTINUED

To make the tacos

1. In a medium pot over high heat, combine the lentils and water. Bring to a boil. Reduce the heat to maintain a simmer and cook for 15 minutes. The lentils should be soft. Drain. Transfer to a medium bowl.

2. While the lentils cook, in a small pot, combine the sweet potato and enough water to completely submerge it. Place the pot over high heat and bring to a boil. Cook for about 10 minutes, until soft, then drain and transfer to the bowl with the lentils.

3. Add the oil and taco seasoning to the lentils and sweet potato and stir to incorporate. Taste and add more seasoning, if needed.

To make the guacamole

4. In a medium bowl, stir together the onion, cilantro, lime juice, jalapeño, and salt.

5. In a small bowl, smash the avocado with a fork, keeping it lumpy. Add the avocado to the other ingredients and mix just enough to incorporate the avocado.

To make the pico de gallo

6. In a small bowl, stir together the tomato, onion, cilantro, jalapeño, and salt to taste.

To assemble the tacos

7. Fill the taco shells with the lentil and sweet potato mixture. Top with Cheddar cheese, sour cream, guacamole, and pico de gallo, as desired.

Make-ahead tip: If you're making sweet potatoes, make extra and refrigerate for up to 3 days. If making this dish with sweet potatoes and lentils cooked ahead, heat the oil in a skillet over medium heat, add the cooked, cooled lentils, sweet potato, and taco seasoning, and stir to combine until heated through.

Per Serving: Calories: 549; Total Fat: 26g; Total Carbs: 61g; Fiber: 12g; Sugar: 5g; Protein 20g; Sodium: 441mg

Summery Butter Bean Soup with Fresh Parsley and Mint

Prep time: 15 minutes / **Cook time:** 20 minutes, plus 10 minutes to infuse the herbs
Serves: 4
Clean Eating, Low-Calorie, Low-Fat, One Pot

Butter beans, or lima beans, have a buttery texture and blend well in summery fare like this Lebanese-inspired soup. Other beans, like kidney beans, work well in hearty chilis and other cold-weather dishes. Butter beans have 7 grams of fiber for every 3½-ounce serving, which includes soluble fiber, especially beneficial for a slow rise in blood sugar.

4 cups vegetable
    broth, divided
1 onion, chopped
2 celery stalks, chopped
1 carrot, chopped
1 leek, rinsed well
    and chopped
2 garlic cloves, minced
5 artichoke
    hearts, chopped
1 (14-ounce) can butter
    beans, drained
    and rinsed
½ teaspoon dried oregano
¾ to 1 teaspoon salt
Freshly ground
    black pepper
¼ cup finely chopped fresh
    mint leaves
¼ cup finely chopped
    fresh parsley

1. In a large pot over medium heat, combine 2 tablespoons of broth, the onion, celery, carrot, and leek. Cook for about 5 minutes, stirring occasionally, until the mixture softens. If the broth cooks off, add more and use it to deglaze the pan, scraping up any browned bits stuck to the bottom.

2. Add the garlic, reduce the heat to low, and cook for 2 to 3 minutes, until softened.

3. Add the artichoke hearts, butter beans, oregano, and remaining broth. Bring to a low boil. Simmer for 10 minutes to let the flavors blend.

4. Taste and season with salt and pepper. Turn off the heat and stir in the mint and parsley to incorporate. Let sit for 10 minutes so the herbs infuse the soup with their flavor.

Addition tip: Serve with Salmon Sandwich with Black Olives and Red Onion (page 146).

Per Serving: Calories: 159; Total Fat: 1g; Total Carbs: 31g; Fiber: 7g; Sugar: 6g; Protein 7g; Sodium: 1173mg

Vegetarian Chili with Cranberries

Prep time: 10 minutes / **Cook time:** 30 minutes
Serves: 6
Clean Eating, Low-Fat, One Pot

The pizzazz with this chili is the cranberries. Everyone who tastes it tells me what a great addition they are. I use frozen cranberries and they thaw quickly after just a couple of minutes in the hot chili. This tart fruit has more than 10 percent of your daily requirement for vitamin C, manganese, and fiber in a 3½-ounce serving.

1 tablespoon extra-virgin olive oil, high-oleic sunflower oil, safflower oil, or canola oil

1 small onion, chopped

1 celery stalk, chopped

1 carrot, chopped

1 garlic clove, minced

2 tablespoons chili powder

1 teaspoon red pepper flakes

1 (28-ounce) can stewed tomatoes, with liquid

1 (14-ounce) can red kidney beans, drained and rinsed

1 cup fresh or frozen cranberries

2 tablespoons chopped fresh parsley

1. In a large pot over medium heat, heat the oil. Add the onion, celery, and carrot. Cook for about 8 minutes, stirring, until tender. Stir in the garlic, chili powder, and red pepper flakes to combine. Reduce the heat to medium-low and cook for about 3 minutes to soften the garlic.

2. Pour the liquid from the tomatoes into the pot. Use an immersion blender to cut through the tomato pieces in the can, leaving some texture, if desired. Add the tomatoes to the pot along with the kidney beans. Increase the heat to medium and bring the chili to a simmer. Cook for about 15 minutes to let the flavors develop.

3. Stir in the cranberries and cook for 2 to 3 minutes to incorporate the flavors.

4. Sprinkle with fresh parsley just before serving.

Variation tip: For more protein, add 1 pound of cooked ground chicken, turkey, beef, or sausage. To keep it vegetarian, add veggie ground round, textured vegetable protein, or a second variety of beans, such as black beans.

Per Serving: Calories: 138; Total Fat: 3g; Total Carbs: 23g; Fiber: 6g; Sugar: 7g; Protein 6g; Sodium: 525mg

Quick Lentil Curry with Sweet Potatoes

Prep time: 15 minutes / **Cook time:** 30 minutes
Serves: 6
Clean Eating, Low-Fat, One Pot

I love how quickly this recipe comes together and that it has so many great things going for it. Sweet potatoes and carrots are high in beta-carotene, and lentils are a good vegetarian protein source. The spices in the curry paste (I use Patak's brand Madras flavor) also add to the health benefits of this dish. If the curry is too spicy for you, use a generous amount of yogurt to help cool the heat.

1 cup lentils, rinsed

1 tablespoon extra-virgin olive oil

1 small yellow onion, chopped

1 carrot, chopped

1 garlic clove, minced

1 tablespoon curry paste

4 cups vegetable broth

1 sweet potato, peeled and chopped

½ cup unsweetened plain yogurt (optional)

1 tablespoon chopped fresh cilantro (optional)

1. In a medium bowl, combine the lentils with enough water to cover by 2 inches or more. Let soak until needed.

2. In a large pot over medium heat, heat the oil. Add the onion and carrot and cook for 4 to 6 minutes, stirring, until softened.

3. Add the garlic and reduce the heat to low. Cook for about 3 minutes, stirring, until soft. Stir in the curry paste.

4. Add the vegetable broth and sweet potato, increase the heat to high, and bring the mixture to a boil. Reduce the heat to a simmer and cook for about 10 minutes, or until the sweet potato is soft enough to puree with an immersion blender.

5. Using an immersion blender, puree half to three-fourths of the sweet potato to create a creamy consistency.

6. Drain the soaking lentils and add them to the pot. Cook for about 10 minutes, until soft.

7. Serve topped with yogurt (if using) and cilantro (if using).

Make-ahead tip: This curry keeps well refrigerated in an airtight container for several days.

Per Serving: Calories: 177; Total Fat: 3g; Total Carbs: 29g; Fiber: 5g; Sugar: 4g; Protein 9g; Sodium: 453mg

Salmon Sandwich with Black Olives and Red Onion

Prep time: 10 minutes

Serves: 2

5 Ingredients or Less, 30 Minutes or Less, Clean Eating

Salmon in a can is generally from wild, not farmed, sources, which makes many consumers feel better about purchasing it. In addition to being an excellent source of anti-inflammatory omega-3 fatty acids, salmon can be a source of calcium if you incorporate the small, edible bones. Enjoy this savory, colorful sandwich with a salad or soup.

1 (6-ounce) can salmon, drained, skin and large bones removed, small bones smashed into the flesh

1 tablespoon minced red onion

1 tablespoon chopped pitted black olives

2 tablespoons mayonnaise

4 slices whole-grain bread

In a medium bowl, stir together the salmon, red onion, olives, and mayonnaise. Divide the salmon mixture evenly between 2 slices of bread. Top with the remaining 2 slices of bread and serve.

Variation tip: For a low-carb wrap version, wrap the salmon filling in collard greens or lettuce leaves. If you want a salad plate, substitute this salmon for the tuna in the Mediterranean Salad Plate (page 104).

Per Serving: Calories: 434; Total Fat: 19g; Total Carbs: 37g; Fiber: 6g; Sugar: 6g; Protein 28g; Sodium: 718mg

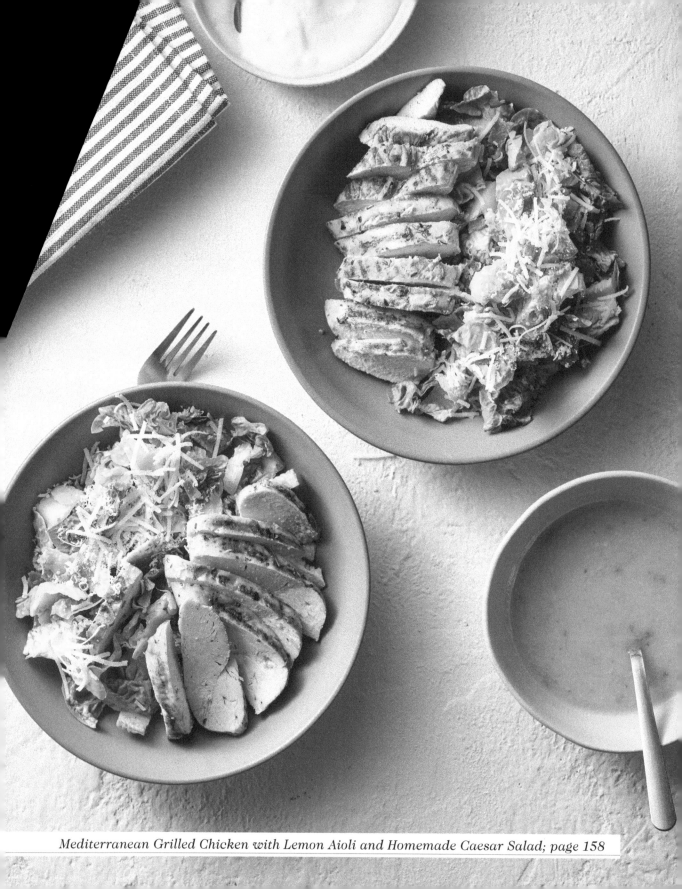

Mediterranean Grilled Chicken with Lemon Aioli and Homemade Caesar Salad; page 158

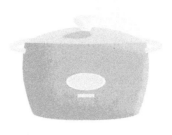

CHAPTER TWELVE

Keto Recipes

Some people start with the keto diet and move to intermittent fasting; others do it in the opposite order. Keeping keto while fasting may help accelerate fat burning and reductions in glucose and insulin, but it's not a necessary part of IF.

Breakfast Sandwich with Jalapeño Keto Mug Bread

Prep time: 10 minutes / **Cook time:** 15 minutes
Serves: 2
30 Minutes or Less, Keto, Low-Carb

Almond flour is lower in carbohydrates and higher in fat than wheat flour and can be used in keto baking. This keto mug bread cooks in 90 seconds in the microwave and is a moist bread that resembles toast when fried. It can be flavored to complement the meal. In this recipe, we'll use jalapeño to do so.

7 tablespoons
butter, divided

3 large eggs, divided

5 tablespoons heavy
(whipping) cream,
divided

1 teaspoon baking powder

⅛ teaspoon salt

6 tablespoons super-
fine almond flour
(no almond skins)

½ teaspoon finely diced
jalapeño pepper

1 teaspoon finely minced
fresh chives (optional)

2 breakfast sausage
patties, cooked

1. Put 1 tablespoon of butter in each of 2 similar-size microwave-safe mugs. Melt the butter for about 20 seconds on high power in the microwave. Swirl the mug to coat the sides with the melted butter.

2. In a small bowl, whisk 1 egg, 3 tablespoons of heavy cream, the baking powder, salt, almond flour, and jalapeño to blend. Evenly divide the batter between the buttered mugs. Microwave on high power for 90 seconds. Let sit for 1 minute. Remove the bread from the mugs and cut each "loaf" horizontally into 2 round bread disks.

3. In a skillet over medium heat, melt 2 tablespoons of butter. Add the bread disks and fry for about 2 minutes, until brown and toasty on one side. Flip the bread, add 2 tablespoons of butter to the skillet, and fry for about 2 minutes more, until brown on the other side. Remove and set aside.

4. In a small bowl, whisk the remaining 2 eggs, remaining 2 tablespoons of heavy cream, and the chives (if using).

5. Add the remaining 1 tablespoon of butter to the skillet and place it over medium heat. Pour in the egg mixture. Cover and cook for about 5 minutes until no longer liquid.

6. Place one slice of toasted keto mug bread on a plate, add 1 cooked sausage and half the scrambled eggs. Top with a second slice of toasted bread. Repeat for the second sandwich.

Variation tip: Instead of jalapeño pepper, try these flavor combinations for your mug bread: 2 black olives, minced and ¼ teaspoon of dried rosemary leaves, crumbled or 2 black olives, minced, and 1 teaspoon of minced sun-dried tomato.

Per Serving: Calories: 890; Total Fat: 86g; Total Carbs: 7g; Fiber: 2g; Sugar: 3g; Protein 26g; Sodium: 1156mg

Spicy Keto Chicken Tenders with Parmesan Mayo

Prep time: 20 minutes / **Cook time:** 20 minutes
Serves: 4
Keto, Low-Carb

These chicken tenders might look like kid's food, but the chipotle chile powder elevates this dish for the adult palate. Almond flour helps keep the carb level down and adds calcium and vitamin E. This might become your favorite way to eat chicken strips.

For the chicken

1 large egg

1 tablespoon heavy (whipping) cream

⅔ cup superfine almond flour (without almond skins)

¼ cup full-fat grated Parmesan cheese

1 teaspoon freshly ground black pepper

1 teaspoon chipotle chile powder

12 ounces boneless, skinless chicken breast, cut into strips

1 cup high-oleic sunflower oil, safflower oil, or canola oil

To make the chicken

1. In a small bowl, whisk together the egg and heavy cream. Set aside.

2. In another small bowl, stir together the almond flour, Parmesan cheese, black pepper, and chipotle powder to combine.

3. Working with one piece at a time, dip the chicken into the flour dredge, then the egg mixture, and into the flour dredge again.

4. In an electric skillet set to 350°F or in a skillet over medium-high heat on the stovetop, heat the oil. To test that the oil is hot enough, dip the handle of a wooden spoon in it; if the oil bubbles around the spoon, it's ready.

5. Working in batches, carefully add the battered chicken to the hot oil. Cook for about 4 minutes until golden brown. Flip and cook for about 4 minutes more, until golden on the other side.

To make the Parmesan mayo

6. While the chicken cooks, in a small bowl, stir together the mayonnaise, Parmesan cheese, garlic powder, and onion flakes. Set aside.

7. Serve the fried chicken with the Parmesan mayo.

Addition tip: Serve with a salad or low-carbohydrate vegetable.

Per Serving: Calories: 607; Total Fat: 54g; Total Carbs: 6g; Fiber: 2g; Sugar: 1g; Protein 27g; Sodium: 285mg

For the Parmesan mayo

¼ cup full-fat mayonnaise

1 tablespoon full-fat grated Parmesan cheese

¼ teaspoon garlic powder

¼ teaspoon onion flakes

Creamy and Delicious Keto Clam Chowder

Prep time: 15 minutes / **Cook time:** 20 minutes
Serves: 4
Keto, Low-Carb

Clams are an excellent source of protein, iron, zinc, selenium, and vitamin B_{12}. This recipe may taste like a gourmet restaurant soup, but it's easy and relatively quick to make! Unlike other soups that need to simmer for a long time, once the vegetables are softened, this soup has a short simmer time.

4 bacon slices, chopped
2 tablespoons butter
1 small onion, finely chopped (⅓ cup)
1 celery stalk, finely chopped
1 (8-ounce) jar clam juice, divided
1 garlic clove, minced
2 tablespoons coconut flour or fine almond flour
1 (14-ounce) can baby clams, drained
1 cup heavy (whipping) cream
½ teaspoon salt
8 thyme sprigs
2 tablespoons chopped fresh parsley
Freshly ground black pepper

1. In a large pot over medium heat, cook the bacon for 5 to 7 minutes, until crispy, then transfer to a plate. Leave the bacon drippings in the pot.

2. Add the butter, onion, and celery to the pot with the drippings and cook over medium heat for about 5 minutes, until softened. Add 2 tablespoons of clam juice to deglaze the pot, scraping the cooked bacon bits from the bottom of the pot. Add the garlic and reduce the heat to medium-low.

3. Stir in the remaining clam juice and coconut flour until the mixture thickens.

4. Add the baby clams, heavy cream, salt, thyme, and parsley. Cook for 3 to 5 minutes to heat through. Taste and season with pepper as desired. Serve in 4 bowls and add the crumbled bacon on top.

Variation tip: If you want to enjoy the chowder with bread, make keto mug bread (page 150).

Per Serving: Calories: 399; Total Fat: 32g; Total Carbs: 7g; Fiber: 2g; Sugar: 3g; Protein 22g; Sodium: 1152mg

Beef Kebabs with Avocado Aioli and Summer Salad

Prep time: 20 minutes / **Cook time:** 20 minutes
Serves: 4
Keto, Low-Carb

Beef is an excellent source of vitamin B$_{12}$, niacin, selenium, zinc, and protein. To keep this meal keto, use low-carb vegetables and wrap the beef in bacon. It comes with a side of aioli, too, for a delicious meal that will leave you feeling satisfied for a long time. Marinating the meat in antioxidant-rich spices and olive oil and cooking over indirect heat can help reduce the formation of carcinogens when you grill. If you choose to use wooden skewers for your kebabs, make sure you soak them in water for at least 20 minutes to prevent burning.

For the aioli

1 large avocado, halved, pitted, peeled, and smashed
¼ cup full-fat mayonnaise
2 garlic cloves, minced

For the beef

3 garlic cloves, minced
¼ cup extra-virgin olive oil
½ teaspoon dried rosemary
¼ teaspoon dried oregano
¼ teaspoon dried basil
⅛ teaspoon freshly ground black pepper
1¼ pounds beef sirloin tip roast, cut into 16 large chunks (4 per skewer)
4 bacon slices, halved widthwise (2 per skewer)

For the vegetables

1 tablespoon extra-virgin olive oil
1 tablespoon grated Parmesan cheese
¼ teaspoon dried basil
¼ teaspoon dried oregano
1 zucchini, cut into 8 large pieces (2 per skewer)
8 mushrooms (2 per skewer)

CONTINUED

To make the aioli

1. In a medium bowl, gently stir together the smashed avocado, mayonnaise, and garlic. Set aside.

To make the beef

2. In a large bowl, whisk together the garlic, oil, rosemary, oregano, basil, and pepper to combine. Add the beef chunks and gently toss to coat. Let sit while you prepare the vegetables.

To make the vegetables

3. In a medium bowl, whisk together the oil, Parmesan, basil, and oregano to blend. Add the zucchini and mushrooms and stir to coat. Let sit.

To assemble the kebabs

4. Wrap 1 piece of beef with ½ bacon slice and place it on a skewer to hold the bacon in place. Add 1 mushroom, 1 zucchini piece, 2 pieces of beef (not wrapped in bacon), 1 mushroom, 1 zucchini piece, and a piece of beef wrapped with ½ bacon slice, so only the outside pieces of meat have bacon. Repeat with the remaining 3 skewers.

5. Preheat the grill: Turn off the heat in the middle section of the grill and turn the surrounding sections to medium heat.

6. Place the skewers over the middle section, without heat. Close the lid and cook for about 16 minutes, flipping the kebabs a quarter turn every 4 minutes, until they are cooked to your desired doneness.

7. Serve with a low-carb side salad, if desired, and use the aioli as a thick salad dressing and dip to dunk your meat and grilled vegetables into.

Variation tip: Cook the kebabs in your oven's broiler for about 16 minutes, turning them every 4 or 5 minutes until cooked through, watching to make sure they don't burn.

Per Serving (1 kebab with aioli): Calories: 623; Total Fat: 50g; Total Carbs: 9g; Fiber: 5g; Sugar:3 g; Protein 35g; Sodium: 334mg

Mediterranean Grilled Chicken with Lemon Aioli and Homemade Caesar Salad

Prep time: 35 minutes / **Cook time:** 15 minutes
Serves: 2
Keto, Low-Carb

There are ways to minimize the formation of carcinogens when meat is cooked at high temperatures or over a flame. By marinating the meat in antioxidant-rich ingredients (olive oil, lemon juice, garlic, oregano, and rosemary), you minimize the formation of these compounds. It's protective to not cook directly over the flame. This is a delicious way to enjoy grilled chicken.

For the chicken

- 3 tablespoons extra-virgin olive oil
- 3 tablespoons freshly squeezed lemon juice
- 1 garlic clove, minced
- 1 teaspoon dried rosemary, crushed
- ½ teaspoon dried oregano
- ¼ teaspoon salt
- ¼ teaspoon freshly ground black pepper
- 2 (4-ounce) boneless, skinless chicken breasts

For the aioli

- ½ cup full-fat mayonnaise
- 1 garlic clove, crushed
- 4 teaspoons freshly squeezed lemon juice

For the salad

- 2 large egg yolks (see tip)
- 3 tablespoons grated full-fat Parmesan cheese
- 2 tablespoons extra-virgin olive oil
- 2 tablespoons freshly squeezed lemon juice, plus more as needed
- 2 anchovy fillets, finely chopped
- ¼ teaspoon Worcestershire sauce, plus more as needed
- ⅛ teaspoon garlic powder, plus more as needed
- 4 cups torn romaine lettuce pieces
- 3 bacon slices, cooked and crumbled

To make the chicken

1. In a large bowl, whisk together the oil, lemon juice, garlic, rosemary, oregano, salt, and pepper to blend.

2. Make ¼-inch-deep cuts into the chicken breasts about 1 inch apart. Place the chicken breasts in the marinade and turn to coat. Let marinate at room temperature for at least 20 minutes, or up to several hours in the refrigerator.

To make the aioli

3. In a small bowl, stir together the mayonnaise, garlic, and lemon juice. Cover and refrigerate until needed.

To make the salad

4. In a large bowl, whisk together the egg yolks, Parmesan cheese, oil, lemon juice, anchovies, Worcestershire sauce, and garlic powder until smooth. Taste and adjust the seasonings, as desired. Add the lettuce and bacon and toss to coat and combine.

5. Preheat the grill: Turn off the heat in the center section of the grill and turn the other sections to medium heat.

CONTINUED

6. Remove the chicken from the marinade and place it over the middle section, without heat. Cook for 5 to 7 minutes per side, until the chicken is cooked through and the juices run clear.

7. Alternatively, if you don't have a grill, preheat the oven to 350°F. Bake the chicken for 25 to 30 minutes, or until the chicken's internal temperature reaches 165°F.

8. Serve the chicken with the Caesar salad on the side and lemon aioli for dipping.

Ingredient tip: Be sure to choose eggs without visible cracks. Raw eggs are not recommended for pregnant women, young children, or people who are immunocompromised.

Per Serving: Calories: 984; Total Fat: 89g; Total Carbs: 11g; Fiber: 3g; Sugar: 3g; Protein 37g; Sodium: 1223mg

Fish Curry with Cauliflower Rice

Prep time: 20 minutes / **Cook time:** 15 minutes
Serves: 4
Keto, Low-Carb

I used to reserve ordering curry for when I visited restaurants, because I thought it was too difficult to make at home. But this recipe couldn't be easier and more delicious, thanks to that little bottle of green curry paste. This is a restaurant-quality meal that you can easily make at home.

12 ounces white fish, such as bass, halibut, or sole
Salt
Freshly ground black pepper
1 (14-ounce) can full-fat coconut milk
2 tablespoons green Thai curry paste
2 tablespoons chopped fresh cilantro, plus more for garnish (optional)
1 small head cauliflower, washed, leaves removed, head broken into florets
4 tablespoons butter

1. Preheat the oven to 375°F.

2. Season the fish with salt and pepper and place it in a baking dish.

3. In a small bowl, whisk together the coconut milk, curry paste, and cilantro to blend. Pour the liquid over the fish.

4. Bake for about 20 minutes, or until the fish flakes easily with a fork.

5. While the fish bakes, in a food processor, process the cauliflower just until it's the size of rice.

6. In a large pan over medium heat, melt the butter. Add the cauliflower, cover the pan, and cook for 5 to 8 minutes, or until your desired doneness. Taste and season with salt, as desired.

7. Serve the cauliflower rice in shallow bowls and top with the fish and curry sauce. Garnish with fresh cilantro (if using).

Variation tip: For a different flavor, use yellow or red curry paste.

Per Serving: Calories: 320; Total Fat: 30g; Total Carbs: 10g; Fiber: 2g; Sugar: 6g; Protein 19g; Sodium: 344mg

Keto Cauliflower Sushi

Prep time: 20 minutes / **Cook time:** 10 minutes
Serves: 4
30 Minutes or Less, Keto, Low-Carb

If you've never rolled your own sushi before, don't be scared to try this. In fact, using the cauliflower rice mixed with avocado makes this sushi an easy texture to roll. There is one trick though, which is cutting the roll into pieces. You need a sharp knife for this or else the contents will squish out of the end. If you don't have a sharp knife, try using a serrated knife to gently cut through the sushi roll. This is a recipe that kids will love to help with!

1 (1- to 2-inch) piece fresh
  ginger, peeled and thinly
  sliced, or pickled ginger

Juice of 1 lemon

1 small head cauliflower,
  leaves removed, head cut
  into florets

2 avocados, halved, pitted,
  and peeled; 1 mashed,
  1 thinly sliced

1 teaspoon wasabi powder
  or paste

4 to 6 nori sheets

2 ounces smoked salmon,
  cut in ½-inch strips

1 cucumber, thinly sliced
  into long strips (optional)

Wasabi mustard,
  for serving

Soy sauce or tamari,
  for serving

1. Preheat the oven to 400°F.

2. In a small bowl, combine the ginger slices and lemon juice. Set aside.

3. In a food processor, process the cauliflower just until it's the size of rice. Spread the cauliflower on a baking sheet.

4. Bake for 8 to 10 minutes, until steamy and moist. Let cool for 5 to 10 minutes. Transfer to a medium bowl.

5. Add the mashed avocado to the cauliflower rice, a little at a time, and mix just until the cauliflower has a sticky consistency. Add the wasabi and adjust to taste.

6. Place 1 nori sheet on a bamboo sushi roller or aluminum foil. Spread one-fourth to one-sixth of the cauliflower-avocado-wasabi mixture in a thin uniform layer over the nori sheet, leaving a ¾-inch margin at the top of the sheet.

7. At the end closest to you, place one-quarter of the salmon slices across the width of the nori sheet. Top with one-quarter of the total avocado slices and cucumber slices (if using).

8. Gently roll up the nori sheet into a sushi roll. Repeat with the remaining nori sheets and remaining filling and ingredients.

9. Let the rolls sit for about 10 minutes before slicing. Serve with the lemon-soaked ginger, wasabi mustard, and soy sauce.

Variation tip: To create a fusion between sushi and a salmon smear:

1. Mix the roasted cauliflower rice with about 8 tablespoons of cream cheese, or enough to get the desired consistency to stick to the nori sheet. Add about 4 teaspoons of freshly squeezed lemon juice, taste, and adjust.

2. Add to the nori sheet as directed.

3. Add smoked salmon or lox and sliced avocado. Place 1 caper about every ½ inch or the distance that allows each piece of sushi you cut to contain 1 caper. Sprinkle with fresh dill and paper-thin slices of red onion (optional). Roll up the nori as directed.

4. Serve with thin slices of the lemon-soaked ginger.

Per Serving: Calories: 160; Total Fat: 11g; Total Carbs: 11g; Fiber: 7g; Sugar: 2g; Protein 6g; Sodium: 135mg

Sausage-Stuffed Peppers

Prep time: 15 minutes / **Cook time:** 45 minutes
Serves: 4
Keto, Low-Carb

Hot Italian sausage adds a lot of flavor to this dish, so I don't include too many additional spices. Peppers are a low-carb vegetable with lots of flavor—they're also the best source of vitamin C. In addition, peppers contain vitamins A, B_6, E, and K, potassium, and folate. They are also rich in pigments from the carotenoid family, credited with cancer-fighting abilities.

2 large red bell peppers

2 tablespoons extra-virgin olive oil

1 small onion, chopped

1 celery stalk, finely chopped

12 ounces raw hot Italian sausage, removed from the casings

8 tablespoons full-fat cream cheese, at room temperature

8 tablespoons grated full-fat mozzarella cheese

1. Preheat the oven to 375°F.

2. Halve the red bell peppers from top to bottom. Remove the ribs and seeds. Cut 1 slice off each half and finely chop. Set aside. Place the pepper halves, cut-side up, in a baking dish. Set aside.

3. In a large saucepan over medium heat, heat the oil. Add the onion, celery, and chopped red pepper. Sauté for 5 to 8 minutes, until soft.

4. Chop the sausage and add the meat to the pan. Stir to incorporate. Cook for about 8 minutes, or until no redness is visible. Turn off the heat and stir in the cream cheese to blend.

5. Divide the mixture into 4 equal parts and spoon into the red pepper halves. Cover each with 2 tablespoons of grated mozzarella cheese.

6. Bake for 30 minutes, or until the cheese is melted and the peppers are soft.

7. Enjoy with a side salad with full-fat dressing.

Variation tip: Try this recipe with your favorite sausage if you prefer something other than hot Italian sausage.

Per Serving: Calories: 511; Total Fat: 43g; Total Carbs: 10g; Fiber: 2g; Sugar: 7g; Protein 22g; Sodium: 885mg

Keto Meatballs with Zucchini Pasta in Tomato Cream Sauce

Prep time: 30 minutes / **Cook time:** 15 minutes
Serves: 4
Keto, Low-Carb

Before creating this recipe, my family didn't eat much red meat or bacon, I never made tomato cream sauce, and my daughter insisted she didn't like pasta. This recipe was a real meal changer for us. We all love these decadent meatballs and tomato cream sauce, and we are now devoted zucchini pasta lovers. This recipe might just change your life, too!

For the meatballs

- 8 ounces ground beef
- 2 bacon slices, cut into small pieces
- 1 large egg
- ¼ cup full-fat grated mozzarella cheese
- ½ small onion, finely diced
- 2 garlic cloves, minced
- 1 tablespoon minced fresh parsley
- 1 tablespoon grated full-fat Parmesan cheese
- 1 teaspoon dried basil
- 1 teaspoon dried oregano
- ½ teaspoon freshly ground black pepper
- 2 tablespoons extra-virgin olive oil

For the sauce

- 1 tablespoon extra-virgin olive oil
- ½ onion, finely diced
- 2 garlic cloves, minced
- 1 cup canned diced tomatoes, with juices
- 2 tablespoons basil pesto
- 1 tablespoon Parmesan cheese, plus more for garnish
- 1 cup heavy (whipping) cream
- ⅛ teaspoon salt
- Fresh parsley, for garnish (optional)
- Red pepper flakes, for seasoning (optional)

For the zucchini pasta

- 2 zucchini, ends removed
- 2 tablespoons extra-virgin olive oil

CONTINUED

To make the meatballs

1. In a large bowl, mix the ground beef, bacon, egg, mozzarella cheese, onion, garlic, parsley, Parmesan cheese, basil, oregano, and pepper. Form the meat mixture into 8 meatballs.

2. In a large skillet over medium-high heat, heat the oil. Add the meatballs. Cook for 4 minutes per side.

To make the sauce

3. In a medium pot over medium heat, heat the oil. Add the onion and sauté for 3 to 4 minutes, until soft. Reduce the heat and add the garlic. Cook for 2 to 3 minutes, stirring frequently.

4. Add the tomatoes and their juices. Use an immersion blender to puree the tomatoes, leaving some texture, if you prefer. Increase the heat and bring the mixture to a simmer. Cook for about 2 minutes.

5. Stir in the pesto, Parmesan cheese, heavy cream, and salt to combine. Reduce the heat to keep warm.

6. Using a vegetable peeler, peel thick strips off the zucchini, including the skin. Continue until you can no longer peel, then cut the remaining core into thin strips. If you have a spiralizer, spiralize the zucchini into noodles.

7. In a large skillet over medium heat, heat the oil. Add the zucchini and pan-fry for about 5 minutes, until soft.

8. Serve the zucchini and meatballs on the plate and top with the tomato cream sauce. Sprinkle with fresh parsley (if using), red pepper flakes (if using), and Parmesan cheese.

Make-ahead tip: Make the meatballs and keep refrigerated for up to 4 hours before cooking.

Per Serving: Calories: 649; Total Fat: 56g; Total Carbs: 15g; Fiber: 3g; Sugar: 8g; Protein 24g; Sodium: 491mg

Creamy Keto Broccoli Soup

Prep time: 20 minutes / **Cook time:** 30 minutes
Serves: 4
Keto, Low-Carb

Broccoli is one of the most nutritious vegetables, packed with fiber, vitamins C and K, folate, and a powerful anti-cancer compound called sulforaphane. For this creamy soup recipe, I use the entire broccoli head, not just the florets.

2 tablespoons extra-virgin olive oil

1 small onion, finely chopped

2 tablespoons butter

2 garlic cloves, minced

1 head broccoli, florets finely chopped and stems peeled and finely grated

2 tablespoons Bone Broth (page 92; optional)

4 cups no-salt-added chicken broth

1 tablespoon cornstarch

⅛ teaspoon cayenne pepper

2 tablespoons grated full-fat Parmesan cheese

2 tablespoons grainy mustard

½ cup heavy (whipping) cream

2 cups grated aged Cheddar cheese

Salt

Freshly ground black pepper

2 tablespoons pumpkin seeds, toasted (optional)

1. In a large pot over medium heat, heat the oil. Add the onion and cook for 5 to 8 minutes to soften. Reduce the heat to medium-low and add the butter and garlic. Cook for 2 to 3 minutes, stirring, until the garlic is soft.

2. Add the broccoli and cook for 3 minutes.

3. Add the bone broth (if using), chicken broth, and cornstarch. Increase the heat to medium-high. Simmer the soup for 10 minutes, until the broccoli is tender.

4. Reduce the heat to medium-low. Stir in the cayenne pepper, Parmesan cheese, mustard, heavy cream, and Cheddar cheese to combine and let the cheese soften and melt.

5. Taste and season with salt and black pepper as needed.

6. Serve topped with the toasted pumpkin seeds (if using).

Variation tip: If full broccoli stalks are too much fiber for you, just use the florets.

Per Serving: Calories: 549; Total Fat: 44g; Total Carbs: 19g; Fiber: 5g; Sugar: 5g; Protein 25g; Sodium: 860mg

Measurement Conversions

VOLUME EQUIVALENTS	U.S. STANDARD	U.S. STANDARD (OUNCES)	METRIC (APPROXIMATE)
LIQUID	2 tablespoons	1 fl. oz.	30 mL
	¼ cup	2 fl. oz.	60 mL
	½ cup	4 fl. oz.	120 mL
	1 cup	8 fl. oz.	240 mL
	1½ cups	12 fl. oz.	355 mL
	2 cups or 1 pint	16 fl. oz.	475 mL
	4 cups or 1 quart	32 fl. oz.	1 L
	1 gallon	128 fl. oz.	4 L
DRY	⅛ teaspoon	–	0.5 mL
	¼ teaspoon	–	1 mL
	½ teaspoon	–	2 mL
	¾ teaspoon	–	4 mL
	1 teaspoon	–	5 mL
	1 tablespoon	–	15 mL
	¼ cup	–	59 mL
	⅓ cup	–	79 mL
	½ cup	–	118 mL
	⅔ cup	–	156 mL
	¾ cup	–	177 mL
	1 cup	–	235 mL
	2 cups or 1 pint	–	475 mL
	3 cups	–	700 mL
	4 cups or 1 quart	–	1 L
	½ gallon	–	2 L
	1 gallon	–	4 L

OVEN TEMPERATURES

FAHRENHEIT	CELSIUS (APPROXIMATE)
250°F	120°C
300°F	150°C
325°F	165°C
350°F	180°C
375°F	190°C
400°F	200°C
425°F	220°C
450°F	230°C

WEIGHT EQUIVALENTS

U.S. STANDARD	METRIC (APPROXIMATE)
½ ounce	15 g
1 ounce	30 g
2 ounces	60 g
4 ounces	115 g
8 ounces	225 g
12 ounces	340 g
16 ounces or 1 pound	455 g

Resources

Online Support

Delay Don't Deny: Intermittent Fasting Support
Facebook.com/groups/DelayDontDeny/

Intermittent Fasting for Women
Facebook.com/groups/510573455951130/members/

Intermittent Fasting for Women Over 40
Facebook.com/groups/227388337812137/

Relevant Articles

American Heart Association. "Is Fasting a Diet Solution?"—This article
reports on inflammation, weight loss, and hunger, and the AHA gives fasting
the green light.
NewsArchive.Heart.org/news/is-fasting-a-diet-solution/

Cleveland Clinic: Health Essentials. "Intermittent Fasting: 4 Different Types
Explained."—This article discusses four different types of intermittent fasting.
Health.ClevelandClinic.org/intermittent-fasting-4-different-types-explained/

Fung, J. "Intermittent Fasting for Beginners."—A series of articles by Dr.
Jason Fung about his use of intermittent fasting in his medical practice.
DietDoctor.com/intermittent-fasting

Heid, Markham. "What Is Intermittent Fasting and Is It Actually Good for
You?" August 1, 2018. *Time.*—*Time* magazine interviews three prominent
intermittent fasting researchers.
Time.com/5354498/is-intermittent-fasting-healthy/

Johns Hopkins Medicine. "Intermittent Fasting: What Is It, and How Does It
Work?" Johns Hopkins Medicine: Health.—This article discusses the 2019

New England Journal of Medicine publication on intermittent fasting.
HopkinsMedicine.org/health/wellness-and-prevention/intermittent-fasting
-what-is-it-and-how-does-it-work

Longo, Valter. "Fasting: Awakening the Rejuvenation from Within." TedX
talk.—Dr. Valter Longo discusses his research on the benefits of fasting for
life extension.
YouTube.com/watch?v=dVArDzYynYc

National Institutes of Health: US National Library of Medicine. "Clinical
Trials on Intermittent Fasting."—Find out what research is being conducted
on intermittent fasting around the world.
ClinicalTrials.gov/ct2/results?cond=intermittent+fasting&term=&cntry=
&state=&city=&dist=

New York State: Department of Environmental Conservation. "Forest
Bathing: Immerse Yourself in a Forest for Better Health."—This article discusses the benefits that forests have on our health.
http://www.dec.ny.gov/lands/90720.html

Sleep Health Foundation. "Are You A Night Owl or an Early Bird?" Accessed
April 24, 2020.—Questionnaire to help you understand your body clock and
which times of the day are more productive for you, as well as which times
are the best for sleep.
https://sleephabits.net/morningness-eveningness-questionnaire

Tello, Monique. "Intermittent Fasting: Surprising Update." June 29, 2018.
Harvard Health *Publishing*: Harvard Medical School.—This article discusses
the benefits of early time restricted feeding.
Health.Harvard.edu/blog/intermittent-fasting-surprising-update-2018062914156

Wolfram, Taylor. "Investigating Intermittent Fasting." October 4, 2018. *Food
& Nutrition.*—This article discusses weight loss and diabetes with intermit-
tent fasting and caution around pregnancy.
FoodandNutrition.org/from-the-magazine/investigating-intermittent-fasting/

Author Blog Posts

"Intermittent Fasting for Women Over 40"
JeanLaMantia.com/cancer-bites-diet-blog/
intermittent-fasting-for-women-over-40/

"The Role of IF for Cancer Treatment and Prevention"
JeanLaMantia.com/cancer-bites-diet-blog/anti-inflammatory-diet/
JeanLaMantia.com/cancer-bites-diet-blog/lymphedema-diet/
JeanLaMantia.com/cancer-bites-diet-blog/can-i-starve-my-cancer/

"Why I Recommend Extra-Virgin Olive Oil, High-Oleic Sunflower and
Safflower Oil, and Expeller-Pressed Canola Oil for My Recipes"
JeanLaMantia.com/cancer-bites-diet-blog/high-oleic-oil/

References

Chapter One

Åkesson, A., A. Eenfeldt, and J. Fung. "Is Intermittent Fasting A Good Idea When Suffering from Stress?" Accessed July 25, 2020. Last updated May 17, 2017. DietDoctor.com/would-you-still-recommend-intermittent-fasting-if-i-have-adrenal-dysfunction.

Berg, J. M., J. L. Tymoczko, and L. Stryer. *Biochemistry*. 5th ed. New York: W. H. Freeman; 2002. Section 30.3, "Food Intake and Starvation Induce Metabolic Changes." Available from: ncbi.nlm.nih.gov/books/NBK22414/.

Bhutani, S., M. C. Klempel, C. M. Kroeger, J. F. Trepanowski, and K. A. Varady. "Alternate Day Fasting and Endurance Exercise Combine to Reduce Body Weight and Favorably Alter Plasma Lipids in Obese Humans." *Obesity* (Silver Spring) 21, no. 7 (July 2013): 1370–9. doi:10.1002/oby.20353.

Carter, S., P. M. Clifton, and J. B. Keogh. "The Effect of Intermittent Compared with Continuous Energy Restriction on Glycaemic Control in Patients with Type 2 Diabetes: 24-Month Follow-Up of a Randomised Noninferiority Trial." *Diabetes Research and Clinical Practice* 151 (2019): 11–19. doi:10.1016/j.diabres.2019.03.022.

Chung, K. W., and H. Y. Chung. "The Effects of Calorie Restriction on Autophagy: Role on Aging Intervention." *Nutrients* 11, no 12 (December 2, 2019): 2923. doi:10.3390/nu11122923.

Clayton, D. J., and L. J. James. "The Effect of Breakfast on Appetite Regulation, Energy Balance, and Exercise Performance." *The Proceedings of the Nutrition Society* 75, no. 3 (August 2016): 319–327. doi:10.1017/S0029665115004243.

de Cabo, Rafael, and Mark P. Mattson. "Effects of Intermittent Fasting on Health, Aging, and Disease." *New England Journal of Medicine* 381, no. (December 26, 2019) [published correction appears in *New England Journal of Medicine* 382, no. 3 (January 16, 2020): 298; correction appears in

New England Journal of Medicine 382, no. 10 (March 5, 2020): 978].
doi:10.1056/NEJMra1905136.

Fung, J. "Fasting and Growth Hormone." Accessed July 26, 2020. Last updated
October 24, 2016. DietDoctor.com/fasting-and-growth-hormone.

Fung, J. "Loose Skin." Last updated May 5, 2017. Accessed June 25, 2020.
YouTube.com/watch?v=5qJeICPLQpk.

Gabel, K., K. K. Hoddy, and K. A. Varady. "Safety of 8-H Time Restricted Feeding in
Adults with Obesity." *Applied Physiology Nutrition and Metabolism* 44, no. 1
(2019): 107–109. doi:10.1139/apnm-2018-0389.

Gibney, M. J., S. I. Barr, F. Bellisle, et al. "Breakfast in Human Nutrition: The International Breakfast Research Initiative." *Nutrients* 10, no 5 (May 2018): 559.
doi:10.3390/nu10050559.

Gill, S., and S Panda. "A Smartphone App Reveals Erratic Diurnal Eating Patterns
in Humans that Can Be Modulated for Health Benefits." *Cell Metabolism* 22,
no. 5 (November 3, 2015): 789–798. doi:10.1016/j.cmet.2015.09.005.

Ho, K. Y., J. D. Veldhuis, M. L. Johnson, et al. "Fasting Enhances Growth Hormone
Secretion and Amplifies the Complex Rhythms of Growth Hormone Secretion
in Man." *The Journal of Clinical Investigation* 81, no 4. (1988): 968–975.
doi:10.1172/JCI113450.

Jamshed, H., R. A. Beyl, D. L. Della Manna, E. S. Yang, E. Ravussin, and C. M.
Peterson. "Early Time-Restricted Feeding Improves 24-Hour Glucose Levels
and Affects Markers of the Circadian Clock, Aging, and Autophagy in Humans."
Nutrients 11, no. 6 (May 30, 2019): 1234. doi:10.3390/nu11061234.

Jovinelly, J., and S. Kim. "Symptoms of Growth Hormone Deficiency." Accessed
June 26, 2020. Last updated January 10, 2019. Healthline.com/health
/growth-hormone-deficiency#symptoms.

Kahleova, H., J. I. Lloren, A. Mashchak, M. Hill, and G. E. Fraser. "Meal Frequency
and Timing Are Associated with Changes in Body Mass Index in Adventist
Health Study 2." *The Journal of Nutrition* 147, no 9 (September 2017):
1722–1728. doi:10.3945/jn.116.244749.

Klempel, M. C., S. Bhutani, M. Fitzgibbon, S. Freels, and K. A. Varady. "Dietary and Physical Activity Adaptations to Alternate Day Modified Fasting: Implications for Optimal Weight Loss." *Nutrition Journal* 9, article no. 35 (September 3, 2010). doi:10.1186/1475-2891-9-35.

Kerndt, P. R., J. L. Naughton, C. E. Driscoll, and D. A. Loxterkamp. "Fasting: The History, Pathophysiology, and Complications." *The Western Journal of Medicine* 137, no. 5 (November1982): 379–99. https://pubmed.ncbi.nlm.nih.gov/6758355/.

López-Sobaler, A. M., E. Cuadrado-Soto, Á. Peral-Suárez, A. Aparicio, and R. M. Ortega. "Importancia del Desayuno en la Mejora Nutricional y Sanitaria de la Población." ["Importance of Breakfast in the Nutritional and Health Improvement of the Population."] *Nutricion Hospitalaria* 35, special no. 6 (September 7, 2018): 3–6. doi:10.20960/nh.2278.

Manoogian, E. N. C., and S. Panda. "Circadian Rhythms, Time-Restricted Feeding, and Healthy Aging." *Ageing Research Reviews* 39 (October 2017):5 9–67. doi:10.1016/j.arr.2016.12.006.

National Institute of Diabetes and Digestive and Kidney Diseases. "Blood Glucose Control Studies for Type 1 Diabetes: DCCT and EDIC." Accessed April 6, 2020. niddk.nih.gov/about-niddk/research-areas/diabetes/blood-glucose-control-studies-type-1-diabetes-dcct-edic.

Rabinowitz, J. D., and E. White. "Autophagy and Metabolism." *Science* 330, no. 6009 (December 3, 2010): 1344–1348. doi:10.1126/science.1193497.

Stote, K. S., D. J. Baer, K. Spears, et al. "A Controlled Trial of Reduced Meal Frequency without Caloric Restriction in Healthy, Normal-Weight, Middle-Aged Adults." The *American Journal of Clinical Nutrition* 85, no. 4 (April *2007*):981–988. doi:10.1093/ajcn/85.4.981.

Welton, S., R. Minty, T. O'Driscoll, et al. "Intermittent Fasting and Weight Loss: Systematic Review." *Canadian Family Physician* 66, no. 2 (February 2020): 117–125. PMID:32060194; PMCID:PMC7021351.

Chapter Two

Bauersfeld, S. P., C. S. Kessler, M. Wischnewsky, et al. "The Effects of Short-Term Fasting on Quality of Life and Tolerance to Chemotherapy in Patients with Breast and Ovarian Cancer: A Randomized Cross-Over Pilot Study." *BMC Cancer* 18, no. 1 (April 27, 2018): 476. doi:10.1186/s12885-018-4353-2.

Chiofalo, B., A. S., Laganà, V. Palmara, et al. "Fasting as Possible Complementary Approach for Polycystic Ovary Syndrome: Hope or Hype?" *Medical Hypotheses* 105 (August 2017): 1–3. doi:10.1016/j.mehy.2017.06.013.

de Cabo, Rafael, and Mark P. Mattson. "Effects of Intermittent Fasting on Health, Aging, and Disease." *New England Journal of Medicine* 381, no. (December 26, 2019) [published correction appears in *New England Journal of Medicine* 382, no. 3 (January 16, 2020): 298; correction appears in *New England Journal of Medicine* 382, no. 10 (March 5, 2020): 978]. doi:10.1056/NEJMra1905136.

de Groot, S., H. Pijl, J. J. M. van der Hoeven, and J. R. Kroep. "Effects of Short-Term Fasting on Cancer Treatment." *Journal of Experimental & Clinical Cancer Research* 38, no. 1 (May 22, 2019): 209. doi:10.1186/s13046-019-1189-9.

Dorff, T. B., S. Groshen, A. Garcia, et al. "Safety and Feasibility of Fasting in Combination with Platinum-Based Chemotherapy." *BMC Cancer* 16, article no. 360 (June 10, 2016). doi:10.1186/s12885-016-2370-6.

Furmli, S., R. Elmasry, M. Ramos, and J. Fung. "Therapeutic Use of Intermittent Fasting for People with Type 2 Diabetes as an Alternative to Insulin." *BMJ Case Reports* 2018 (October 9, 2018). doi:10.1136/bcr-2017-221854.

Gibson, E. M., W. P. Williams 3rd, and L. J. Kriegsfeld. "Aging in the Circadian System: Considerations for Health, Disease Prevention, and Longevity." *Experimental Gerontology* 44, nos. 1–2 (January–February 2009): 51–56. doi:10.1016/j.exger.2008.05.007.

Grajower, M. M., and B. D. Horne. "Clinical Management of Intermittent Fasting in Patients with Diabetes Mellitus." *Nutrients* 11, no. 4 (April 18, 2019): 873. doi:10.3390/nu11040873.

Horne, B. D., H. T. May, J. L. Anderson, et al. "Usefulness of Routine Periodic Fasting to Lower Risk of Coronary Artery Disease in Patients Undergoing Coronary Angiography." *The American Journal of Cardiology* 102, no. 7 (October 2008): 814–819. doi:10.1016/j.amjcard.2008.05.021.

Icard, P., L. Ollivier, P. Forgez, et al. "Perspective: Do Fasting, Caloric Restriction, and Diets Increase Sensitivity to Radiotherapy? A Literature Review." Advances in Nutrition [published online ahead of print] (June 3, 2020). doi:10.1093/advances/nmaa062.

Johnson, J. B., W. Summer, R. G. Cutler, et al. "Alternate Day Calorie Restriction Improves Clinical Findings and Reduces Markers of Oxidative Stress and Inflammation in Overweight Adults with Moderate Asthma." *Free Radical Biology & Medicine* 42, no. 5 (2007): 665–674. doi:10.1016/j.freeradbiomed.2006.12.005.

Longo, V. D., and S. Panda. "Fasting, Circadian Rhythms, and Time-Restricted Feeding in Healthy Lifespan." *Cell Metabolism* 23, no.6 (2016): 1048–1059. doi:10.1016/j.cmet.2016.06.001.

Malinowski, B., K. Zalewska, A. Węsierska, et al. "Intermittent Fasting in Cardiovascular Disorders—An Overview." *Nutrients* 11, no. 3 (March 20, 2019): 673. doi:10.3390/nu11030673.

Marinac, C. R., S. H. Nelson, C. I. Breen, et al. "Prolonged Nightly Fasting and Breast Cancer Prognosis." *JAMA Oncology* 2, no. 8 (2016): 1049–1055. doi:10.1001/jamaoncol.2016.0164.

Moro, T., G. Tinsley, A. Bianco, et al. "Effects of Eight Weeks of Time-Restricted Feeding (16/8) on Basal Metabolism, Maximal Strength, Body Composition, Inflammation, and Cardiovascular Risk doi:10.1186/s12967-016-1044-0Factors in Resistance-Trained Males." *Journal of Translational Medicine* 14, no. 1 (October 13, 2016): 290. doi:10.1186/s12967-016-1044-0.

Müller, H., F. W. de Toledo, and K. L. Resch. "Fasting Followed by Vegetarian Diet in Patients with Rheumatoid Arthritis: A Systematic Review." *Scandinavian Journal of Rheumatology* 30, no. 1 (2001): 1–10. doi:10.1080/030097401750065256.

O'Flanagan, C. H., L. A. Smith, S. B. McDonell, and S. D. Hursting. "When Less May Be More: Calorie Restriction and Response to Cancer Therapy." *BMC Medicine* 15, no. 1 May 24, 2017): 106. doi:10.1186/s12916-017-0873-x.

Rynders, C. A., E. A. Thomas, A. Zaman, Z. Pan, V. A. Catenacci, and E. L. Melanson. "Effectiveness of Intermittent Fasting and Time-Restricted Feeding Compared to Continuous Energy Restriction for Weight Loss." *Nutrients* 11, no. 10 (October 14, 2019):2 442. doi:10.3390/nu11102442.

Safdie, F. M., T. Dorff, D. Quinn, et al. "Fasting and Cancer Treatment in Humans: A Case Series Report." *Aging* 1, no. 12 (December 31, 2009): 988–1007. doi:10.18632/aging.100114.

Santos, H. O., and R. C. O. Macedo. "Impact of Intermittent Fasting on the Lipid Profile: Assessment Associated with Diet and Weight Loss." *Clin Nutrition ESPEN* 24 (2018): 14–21. doi:10.1016/j.clnesp.2018.01.00.2.

Zangeneh, F., R. Salman Yazdi, M. M. Naghizadeh, and N. Abedinia. "Effect of Ramadan Fasting on Stress Neurohormones in Women with Polycystic Ovary Syndrome." *Journal of Family and Reproductive Health* 9, no. 2 (2015): 51–57.

Chapter Three

Fung, J. "Longer Fasting Regimes—24 Hours or More." Accessed April 29, 2020. Last updated October 3, 2016. DietDoctor.com/longer-fasting-regimens.

Galindo Muñoz, J. S., M. Gómez Gallego, I. Díaz Soler, M. C. Barberá Ortega, C. M. Martínez Cáceres, and J. J. Hernández Morante. "Effect of a Chronotype-Adjusted Diet on Weight Loss Effectiveness: A Randomized Clinical Trial." *Clinical Nutrition* 39, no. 4 (April 2020): 1041–1048. doi:10.1016/j.clnu.2019.05.012.

Heilbronn, L. K., S. R. Smith, C. K. Martin, S. D. Anton, and E. Ravussin. "Alternate-Day Fasting in Nonobese Subjects: Effects on Body Weight, Body Composition, and Energy Metabolism." *The American Journal of Clinical Nutrition* 81, no. 1 (January 2005): 69–73. doi:10.1093/ajcn/81.1.69.

LeanGains. "Brief Summary of Popular Approaches to Intermittent Fasting."
Accessed April 15, 2020. Last updated June 19, 2008. LeanGains.com/brief
-summary-of-popular-approaches-to-intermittent-fasting/.

Levy, E., and T. Chu. "Intermittent Fasting and Its Effects on Athletic Performance:
A Review." *Current Sports Medicine Reports* 18, no. 7 (July 2019): 266–269.
doi:10.1249/JSR.0000000000000614.

Paoli, A., G. Tinsley, A. Bianco, and T. Moro. "The Influence of Meal Frequency
and Timing on Health in Humans: The Role of Fasting." *Nutrients* 11, no. 4
(March 28, 2019):7 19. doi:10.3390/nu11040719.

Plowe, K., and C. Thompson C. "The Warrior Diet Might Help You Lose Weight—
but There Are Some Risks to Know." Accessed April 29, 2020. Last updated
June 1, 2020. LiveStrong.com/article/83394-start-warrior-diet/.

Sleep Health Foundation. "Are You A Night Owl or an Early Bird?" Accessed
April 24, 2020. https://www.sleephealthfoundation.org.au/pdfs/World%20
Sleep%20Day/Activity%20-%20Morning-Eveningness%20Questionnaire.pdf.

Sutton, E. F., R. Beyl, K. S. Early, W. T. Cefalu, E. Ravussin, and C. M. Peterson.
"Early Time-Restricted Feeding Improves Insulin Sensitivity, Blood Pressure,
and Oxidative Stress Even without Weight Loss in Men with Prediabetes."
Cell Metabolism 27, no. 6 (June 5, 2018): 1212–1221.e3. doi:10.1016/j.cmet
.2018.04.010.

Chapter Four

American College of Pediatricians. "The Benefits of the Family Table." May 2014.
Accessed May 9, 2020. Last updated May 2014. acpeds.org/position-statements
/the-benefits-of-the-family-table.

Carter, S., P. M. Clifton, and J. B. Keogh. "Effect of Intermittent Compared with
Continuous Energy Restricted Diet on Glycemic Control in Patients with Type
2 Diabetes: A Randomized Noninferiority Trial." *JAMA Network Open* 1, no. 3
(July 6, 2018): e180756. doi:10.1001/jamanetworkopen.2018.0756.

Carter, S., P. M. Clifton PM, and J. B. Keogh. "The Effect of Intermittent Compared
with Continuous Energy Restriction on Glycaemic Control in Patients

with Type 2 Diabetes: 24-Month Follow-Up of a Randomised Noninferiority Trial." *Diabetes Research and Clinical Practice* 151 (May 2019): 11–19. doi:10.1016/j.diabres.2019.03.022.

Catenacci, V. A., Z. Pan Z, D. Ostendorf, et al. "A Randomized Pilot Study Comparing Zero-Calorie Alternate-Day Fasting to Daily Caloric Restriction in Adults with Obesity." *Obesity* (Silver Spring) 24, no. 9 (2016): 1874–1883. doi:10.1002/oby.21581.

Corley, B. T., R. W. Carroll, R. M. Hall, M. Weatherall, A. Parry-Strong, and J. D. Krebs. "Intermittent Fasting in Type 2 Diabetes Mellitus and the Risk of Hypoglycaemia: A Randomized Controlled Trial." *Diabetic Medicine* 35, no. 5 (2018): 588–594. doi:10.1111/dme.13595.

Harvie, M., C. Wright, M. Pegington, et al. "The Effect of Intermittent Energy and Carbohydrate Restriction v. Daily Energy Restriction on Weight Loss and Metabolic Disease Risk Markers in Overweight Women." *The British Journal of Nutrition* 110, no 8 (2013): 1534–1547. doi:10.1017/S0007114513000792.

Higgins, K. A., and R. D. Mattes. "A Randomized Controlled Trial Contrasting the Effects of 4 Low-Calorie Sweeteners and Sucrose on Body Weight in Adults with Overweight or Obesity." *The American Journal of Clinical Nutrition* 109, no. 5 (2019): 1288–1301. doi:10.1093/ajcn/nqy381.

Leidy, H. J., and W. W. Campbell. "The Effect of Eating Frequency on Appetite Control and Food Intake: Brief Synopsis of Controlled Feeding Studies." *The Journal of Nutrition* 141, no. 1 (2011): 154–157. doi:10.3945/jn.109.114389.

Madjd, A., M. A. Taylor, A. Delavari, R. Malekzadeh, I. A. Macdonald, and H. R. Farshchi. "Beneficial Effects of Replacing Diet Beverages with Water on Type 2 Diabetic Obese Women Following a Hypo-Energetic Diet: A Randomized, 24-Week Clinical Trial." *Diabetes, Obesity, and Metabolism* 19, no. 1 (2017): 125–132. doi:10.1111/dom.12793.

Madjd, A., M. A. Taylor, A. Delavari, R. Malekzadeh, I. A. Macdonald, and H. R. Farshchi. "Effects of Replacing Diet Beverages with Water on Weight Loss and Weight Maintenance: 18-Month Follow-Up, Randomized Clinical Trial." *International Journal of Obesity* (London) 42, no. 4 (2018): 835–840. doi:10.1038/ijo.2017.306.

Madjd, A., M. A. Taylor, A. Delavari, R. Malekzadeh, I. A. Macdonald, and H. R. Farshchi. "Effects on Weight Loss in Adults of Replacing Diet Beverages with Water During a Hypoenergetic Diet: A Randomized, 24-Week Clinical Trial." *The American Journal of Clinical Nutrition* 102, no. 6 (2015): 1305–1312. doi:10.3945/ajcn.115.109397.

Pepino, M. Y. "Metabolic Effects of Non-Nutritive Sweeteners." *Physiology and Behavior* 152, Part B (2015): 450–455. doi:10.1016/j.physbeh.2015.06.024.

Pepino, M. Y., C. D. Tiemann, B. W. Patterson, B. M. Wice, and S. Klein. "Sucralose Affects Glycemic and Hormonal Responses to an Oral Glucose Load." *Diabetes Care* 36, no. 9 (2013): 2530–2535. doi:10.2337/dc12-2221.

Rogers, P. J., P. S. Hogenkamp, C. de Graaf, et al. "Does Low-Energy Sweetener Consumption Affect Energy Intake and Body Weight? A Systematic Review, Including Meta-Analyses, of the Evidence from Human and Animal Studies." *International Journal of Obesity* 40, no. 3 (2016): 381–394. doi:10.1038/ijo.2015.177.

Soeters, M. R., N. M. Lammers, P. F. Dubbelhuis, et al. "Intermittent Fasting Does Not Affect Whole-Body Glucose, Lipid, or Protein Metabolism." *The American Journal of Clinical Nutrition* 90, no. 5 (2009): 1244–1251. doi:10.3945/ajcn.2008.27327.

Templeman, I., D. Thompson, J. Gonzalez, et al. "Intermittent Fasting, Energy, Balance, and Associated Health Outcomes in Adults: Study Protocol for a Randomised Controlled Trial." *Trials* 19, no. 1 (February 2, 2018): 86. doi:10.1186/s13063-018-2451-8.

The Fasting Method. "Cephalic Phase Response and Hunger—Phase 18." TheFastingMethod.com/cephalic-phase-response-hunger-fasting-18.

The National Academies of Sciences, Engineering, and Medicine. "Dietary Reference Intakes: Electrolytes and Water." *Dietary Reference Intakes for Water, Potassium, Sodium, Chloride, and Sulfate.* 2004. The National Academies. https://perruchenautomne.eu/wordpress/wp-content/uploads/2014/12/DRI_Electrolytes_Water.pdf.

The National Academies of Sciences, Engineering, and Medicine. "Summary Report of the Dietary Reference Intakes." NationalAcademies.org/our-work/summary-report-of-the-dietary-reference-intakes.

Trepanowski, J. F., C. M. Kroeger, A. Barnosky, et al. "Effect of Alternate-Day Fasting on Weight Loss, Weight Maintenance, and Cardioprotection Among Metabolically Healthy Obese Adults: A Randomized Clinical Trial." *JAMA Internal Medicine* 177, no. 7 (2017): 930–938. doi:10.1001/jamainternmed.2017.0936.

Trepanowski, J. F., C. M. Kroeger, A. Barnosky, et al. "Effects of Alternate-Day Fasting or Daily Calorie Restriction on Body Composition, Fat Distribution, and Circulating Adipokines: Secondary Analysis of a Randomized Controlled Trial." *Clinical Nutrition* 37, no. 6 Part A (2018): 1871–1878. doi:10.1016/j.clnu.2017.11.018.

Varady, K. A., and K. Gabel. "Safety and Efficacy of Alternate Day Fasting." *Nature Reviews. Endocrinology* 15, no. 12 (2019): 686–687. doi:10.1038/s41574-019-0270-y.

Chapter Six

Arciero, P. J., M. I. Goran, and E.T. Poehiman. "Resting Metabolic Rate Is Lower in Women Than in Men." *Journal of Applied Physiology* 75, no. 6 (December 1993): 2514–20.

Centers for Disease Control and Prevention. "Folic Acid." Centers for Disease Control and Prevention. Accessed September 2019. cdc.gov/ncbddd/folicacid/features/folic-acid.html.

De Baaij, J. G., J.G. Hoenderop, and R. J. Bindels. "Magnesium in Man: Implications for Health and Disease." *Physiology Reviews* 95, no. 1 (January 2015): 1–46. https://doi.org/10.1152/physrev.00012.2014.

Harvie, M. N., M. Pegington, M. P. Mattson, J. Frystyk, B. Dillon, G. Evans, et al. "The Effects of Intermittent or Continuous Energy Restriction on Weight Loss and Metabolic Disease Risk Markers: A Randomised Trial in Young Overweight Women." *International Journal of Obesity* 35, no. 5 (October 5, 2010): 714–727.

Chapter Seven

Anton, S., and C. Leeuwenburgh. "Fasting or Caloric Restriction for Healthy Aging." *Experimental Gerontology* 48, no. 10 (October 2013): 1003–1005. doi:10.1016/j.exger.2013.04.011.

Anton, S. D., S. A. Lee, W. T. Donahoo, et al. "The Effects of Time Restricted Feeding on Overweight, Older Adults: A Pilot Study." *Nutrients* 11, no. 7 (June 30 2019): 1500. doi:10.3390/nu11071500.

Everhart, J. E. "Contributions of Obesity and Weight Loss to Gallstone Disease." *Annals of Internal Medicine* 119, no. 10 (November 15, 1993): 1029–1035. doi:10.7326/0003-4819-119-10-199311150-00010.

Gutiérrez, Á., M. González-Gross, M. Delgado, and M. J. Castillo. "Three Days Fast in Sportsmen Decreases Physical Work Capacity but Not Strength or Perception-Reaction Time." *International Journal of Sport Nutrition and Exercise Metabolism* 11, no. 4 (2001): 420–429. doi:10.1123/ijsnem.11.4.420.

Mehler, P. S., A. B., Winkelman, D. M. Andersen, and J. L. Gaudiani. "Nutritional Rehabilitation: Practical Guidelines for Refeeding the Anorectic Patient." *Journal of Nutrition and Metabolism* 2010 (February 7, 2010): 625782. doi:10.1155/2010/625782.

Sakurada, K., T. Konta, M. Watanabe, et al. "Associations of Frequency of Laughter with Risk of All-Cause Mortality and Cardiovascular Disease Incidence in a General Population: Findings from the Yamagata Study." *Journal of Epidemiology* 30, no. 4 (April 2020):188–193. doi:10.2188/jea.JE20180249.

Chapter Eight

Diabetes.co.uk. "Cinnamon and Diabetes." Last updated Jan 15, 2019. Diabetes .co.uk/natural-therapies/cinnamon.html.

Leeman, M., E. Östman, and I. Björck. "Vinegar Dressing and Cold Storage of Potatoes Lowers Postprandial Glycaemic and Insulinaemic Responses in Healthy Subjects." *European Journal of Clinical Nutrition* 59, no. 11 (July 20, 2005): 1266–1271. doi:10.1038/sj.ejcn.1602238.

Chapter Ten

Ayaz, A., A. Akyol, E. Inan-Eroglu, A. Kabasakal Cetin, G. Samur, and F. Akbiyik. "Chia Seed (*Salvia Hispanica L.*) Added Yogurt Reduces Short-Term Food Intake and Increases Satiety: Randomised Controlled Trial." *Nutrition Research and Practice* 11, no. 5 (October 2017): 412–418. doi:10.4162/nrp.2017.11.5.412.

Vuksan, V., A. L. Jenkins, C. Brissette, et al. "Salba-Chia (*Salvia Hispanica L.*) in the Treatment of Overweight and Obese Patients with Type 2 Diabetes: A Double-Blind Randomized Controlled Trial." *Nutrition, Metabolism, and Cardiovascular Diseases* 27, no. 2 (2017): 138–146. doi:10.1016/j.numecd.2016.11.124.

Index

Acknowledgments

I would like to thank Callisto Media for entrusting me with the task of researching, writing, and sharing with the world the very exciting dietary strategy of intermittent fasting. This is my first experience working with Callisto and it's been incredibly positive. I would especially like to thank Susan Lutfi, the acquisitions editor who took the time to explain the project, answered all my questions, and made sure I was comfortable and ready to begin.

It's been a delight from start to finish to be part of the Callisto family. I'd like to thank the executive editor Shannon Robson, who did an excellent job researching—it made my job easier. Thank you to Natasha (Tasha) Yglesias, my managing editor, who worked at lightning speed but was still incredibly thorough, eagle-eyed, and encouraging. Patty Consolazio, my development editor, asked all the right questions to make sure readers would understand every aspect of fasting. Mary Cassells made sure my recipes could be followed, and managing editor Claire Yee helped get this book across the finish line!

Thank you to my kids Leonie and Tatum, who independently finished online school during a pandemic so I could focus on researching and writing. They were great food critics who gave me their honest opinions as I tested all my recipes (Leonie's favorite is Sicilian Eggs and Tatum's is Keto Cauliflower Sushi). I could not have gotten through the recipe development without my friend and next-door neighbor Isabelle Noël, who was always ready to hop over the fence on short notice to taste my recipes. She was a massive help, and I'm grateful for such a great neighbor, especially during such challenging times.

As a registered dietitian for almost three decades, I've seen my share of fad diets. I know it's still early in the research world, but I believe intermittent fasting has the potential to improve the lives of millions of people who desire to lose weight, eliminate type 2 diabetes, improve heart health, reduce cancer risk, and live longer, healthier lives. Along with my professional journey into the world of intermittent fasting, I began my own personal exploration, and I must say, even in the short time I've been doing it, the results have been positive.

I tried intermittent fasting 5:2 and the ketogenic diet about three years ago and personally found it unsustainable. I was hungry and constantly craving and thinking about food. While researching this book, I was inspired by what I read. I experimented with time-restricted feeding this time and found it easy and effective. I point this out so readers know there are many ways and methods to do intermittent fasting. If your first time doesn't work, try something else.

I look forward to using intermittent fasting with my clients to help them improve their health.

About the Author

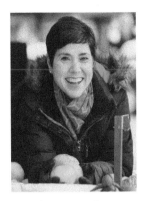

Jean LaMantia, RD, is a registered dietitian with a virtual private practice. She has written two previous books: *The Essential Cancer Treatment Nutrition Guide and Cookbook* and *The Complete Lymphedema Management and Nutrition Guide*. She's also created a food guide for cancer survivors called *The Cancer Risk Reduction Guide*. She's a popular public speaker for topics related to cancer, lymphedema, inflammation, and nutrition and now adds intermittent fasting to her offerings. She uses intermittent fasting in her practice to help clients achieve their goals of weight reduction, reduced inflammation, and improved health. To find out more about Jean and read her *Cancer Bites* blog, visit JeanLaMantia.com.